What's Up
WITH
Your Gut?

This book is dedicated to our families, to Mark, Holly, Annie and Phoebe, and to Ann, and the patients who told us their stories.

What's Up
WITH
Your Gut?

*Why you bloat after eating bread and
pasta... and other gut problems*

Jo Waters
and
Professor Julian Walters

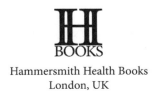

Hammersmith Health Books
London, UK

First published in 2016 by Hammersmith Health Books – an imprint of
Hammersmith Books Limited
4/4A Bloomsbury Square, London WC1A 2RP, UK
www.hammersmithbooks.co.uk

Reprinted 2016

Disclaimer: The information contained in this book is for educational purposes
only. It is the result of the study and the experience of the authors. Whilst the
information and advice offered are believed to be true and accurate at the
time of going to press, neither the authors nor the publisher can accept any
legal responsibility or liability for any errors or omissions that may have been
made or for any adverse effects which may occur as a result of following the
recommendations given herein. Always consult a qualified medical practitioner if
you have any concerns regarding your health.

British Library Cataloguing in Publication Data: A CIP record of this book is
available from the British Library.

Print ISBN 978-1-78161-067-1
Ebook ISBN 978-1-78161-068-8

Commissioning editor: Georgina Bentliff
Copy editor: Carolyn White
Designed and typeset by: Julie Bennett, Bespoke Publishing Ltd.
Cover design by: Sylvia Kwan
Index: Dr Laurence Errington
Production: Helen Whitehorn, Path Projects Ltd.
Printed and bound by: TJ International, UK

Contents

Acknowledgements

We would like to thank the following people and organisations for their help in making this book as thorough as possible.

- NICE (National Institute for Health and Care Excellence) for permission to quote from their Guidelines on irritable bowel syndrome (page 29) and coeliac disease (page 62).
- The Rome Foundation for permission to use the Bristol Stool Chart (page 178).
- Coeliac UK for permission to quote the Marsh Guidelines (page 68).
- The Pelvic Radiation Association for permission to quote their guidance (pages 134-6).
- Dr Kamran Rostami and his patient Sue C for their assistance with the section on non-coeliac gluten sensitivity (pages 72-7).
- The digestive diseases charity Core for background information from its Digesting the Facts report and fact sheets on gut conditions cited as references in chapters 4 (coeliac disease), 6 (Crohn's disease and colitis) and 8 (peptic ulcers and gallstones).
- Crohn's and Colitis UK for background source information for references cited in Chapter 6 on inflammatory bowel diseases.

Preface 1

We are all interested in what we eat, how that makes us what we are, and how we feel about it. Food is a major part of our lives; we eat several times a day and think about eating and our appetites constantly. We have our likes and dislikes, our favourite recipes, cooks and restaurants.

We need our guts to digest and absorb this food. Most of the time, our gastro-intestinal digestive system (the gut) does its job without us being aware of what is going on. We do not spend much of our conscious time thinking about the passage of food from our mouth, through the stomach and intestines, until it comes out the other end. Although we talk about food, we rarely discuss going to the toilet, our bowel habits and what comes out – we have learnt to laugh embarrassedly about 'poo' since we were little.

But we get gut feelings – we know when there is something not quite right – and then want to find out what is going on. Almost all of us have had sickness and vomiting at some time, with belly ache and diarrhoea affecting most people. We then get questions. Was it the food I ate? Have I got these symptoms more than other people? Should I eat differently? Am I ill? Should I go and see a doctor? What about a nutritionist? Will they know what I'm talking about? Is it serious?

In the last few years, there seem to have been more digestive diseases about. Perhaps we are now talking about them more, but maybe we are actually seeing more of these conditions and certainly doctors are much better at making accurate diagnoses – if we know about the latest developments! Several new themes in gut conditions have become popular topics in the last decade or so, with a lot of new ideas flying around. Are these topics, like gluten-free foods, fibre, FODMAPs, bile acids and such, relevant to gut conditions like irritable bowel syndrome (or even cancers), and what should be done about them?

If you have questions like these, I hope this book can help you by providing some facts, explaining recent ideas and providing some answers. Jo Waters writes about health issues in newspapers and magazines, including digestive diseases and related gut conditions, and what to do about them. When we talked about some of these new ideas, we realised it would help to pull them together in a book on your guts.

I hope you find our explanation of these gut topics edifying and something you can digest easily!

Professor Julian Walters
March 2016

Preface 2

I've been fortunate enough to work as a medical journalist for 30 years for the medical trade press, women's magazines and national newspapers – a job I still find totally fascinating. I'm humbled by the stories people tell me about their illnesses and grateful to all the doctors who've been kind enough to spare the time to give me interviews on their areas of expertise.

During dozens of interviews with people suffering from gut complaints over the years though, the stories I heard over and over again were that some people never get an explanation for what is up with their gut. Some are too embarrassed to talk about 'trouble down below' and rely on over-the-counter remedies such as laxatives for constipation or loperamide for diarrhoea – running the risk of ignoring important 'red flag' symptoms for conditions such as inflammatory bowel disease, coeliac disease or even bowel cancer.

Then there are others who experiment with faddy exclusion diets – demonising carbohydrates and cutting out staples like bread and pasta because they're convinced they have gluten sensitivity – but who have never actually been tested for coeliac disease. Those I consider particularly unlucky are those who – for whatever reason – slip through the net and miss out on the tests that could have diagnosed their coeliac disease or cancer much earlier and saved them years of debilitating symptoms and in some cases an early death.

A couple of stories stood out and gave me the impetus to write this book with Professor Julian Walters. The first was interviewing Professor Walters for the *Daily Mail* Good Health section about a condition called BAD – bile acid diarrhoea (also known as BAM – bile acid malabsorption), a cause of a particularly nasty, persistent kind of diarrhoea which can cause up to 10 bowel movements a day and leave people practically housebound. I was staggered when he told me that up to a third of the three million people estimated to have IBS with diarrhoea as the predominant symptom (IBS-D) might have this condition instead, yet hardly anyone has heard of it. Why does it matter? Well, as Professor Walters explained, there's a test for bile acid diarrhoea and an effective treatment. He put me in touch with one of his patients, who emailed him after she'd read about his research. She'd had totally debilitating diarrhoea since her teens and had never got a proper diagnosis or treatment for her symptoms, despite umpteen invasive investigations. After seeing Professor Walters, and having the relevant tests, she was diagnosed with BAD and after 40-odd years of suffering finally got an effective treatment.

Another *Daily Mail* Good Health feature led me to the door of gastroenterolgist Dr Kamran Rostami who wrote up a case report for the *British Medical Journal*. The patient had all the symptoms of coeliac disease but tested negative for it in blood tests and gut biopsies. When he cut out gluten though, his symptoms virtually disappeared. Dr Rostami talked about another condition I'd never heard of called non-coeliac gluten sensitivity (NCGS) and quoted research findings which if applied to the UK population could mean between four and seven million people in total may have this condition. And hardly any one had heard of NCGS either.

After the article was published Dr Rostami received a steady flow of emails from patients wanting to know more about NCGS and the blog I wrote online about NCGS started to get hundreds of views a week. It was then I started to think that maybe there's a need for a book on this – after all, it's estimated three-quarters of people with coeliac disease are still undiagnosed; too many people are still diagnosed with late stage bowel cancer and more and more cancer survivors are being left to deal with pelvic radiation disease – lifelong bowel symptoms caused by cancer treatment. How many more 'hidden' conditions were there? I thought maybe putting all the information about these less well known but surprisngly common conditions together in one place could help more people get to the bottom of what is really up with their gut and get treatment to cure or manage their symptoms.

Now the book has come together and I hope you'll find it a useful steer through all the tests and symptoms that can make diagnosing gut problems such a long drawn-out and sometimes emotionally draining process. It goes without saying that it's not an alternative to seeing a doctor but it may help you along the road to getting a diagnosis. I really hope so.

My sincere thanks go to Professor Julian Walters for his expert guidance and collaboration on this book and, to publisher Georgina Bentliff for her unstinting faith in my original idea and that I would complete this project and to Carolyn White, the editor.

Jo Waters
March 2016

About the Authors

Jo Waters is a health writer for consumer magazines and national newspapers and the co-author of two health books. She is a regular contributor to the *Daily Mail's* weekly Good Health section and a former features editor of *Top Sante* and *Pregnancy & Birth* magazines and also worked as contributing health writer for *Yours* magazine and as news editor for *General Practitioner*. Between 2011 and 2013 she was chair of the Guild of Health Writers.

Julian Walters is Professor of Gastroenterology at Imperial College London, based at the Hammersmith Hospital. As well as teaching medical students and conducting research into the causes of and new treatments for digestive diseases, he sees a wide variety of patients with digestive disorders such as malabsorption and chronic diarrhoea.

Chapter 1

Introduction – what's *really* up with your gut?

This book is written for the millions of people worldwide who suffer from gut problems; from burping and acid reflux to abdominal pain and flatulence through to diarrhoea, bloating, painful cramping and constipation. What happens between eating your food and it coming out the other end can sometimes be a source of daily discomfort and embarrassment.

Whether you bloat after eating pasta, bread or dairy, suffer cramping diarrhoea when you are stressed-out, get constipated when you're on holiday or just feel fatigued by your grumbling guts, we hope it will help you work out how best to manage your symptoms and get appropriate medical help.

These days you can't open a newspaper, click on the internet or attend a dinner party without someone holding court about the latest 'miracle' exclusion diet, where cutting out wheat/gluten/dairy/lactose or sugar has apparently done wonders for their bloating, diarrhoea or grumbling gut pain and usually related weight loss too. In most cases, though, they'll be doing it without consulting their doctor or a dietitian and just hoping for the best, but the danger is they could be cutting out important nutrients and fibre too – plus there's always the risk that there may be a serious underlying medical cause for their symptoms which never gets diagnosed or treated. Critics of exclusion diets say that if symptoms do improve it's more often down to the placebo effect (believing something will work), or just eating less overall, than because of a genuine sensitivity to the excluded food.

This book is an attempt to steer you down the sensible middle road on a route to getting a medical diagnosis and effective treatment for your gut symptoms. It goes without saying it isn't a substitute for seeing your doctor, but if you've had symptoms for a long time and don't seem to be getting anywhere it might give you some really useful pointers for possible causes and/or treatments.

How common are gut problems?

Gut symptoms account for one in five of all GP consultations according to some studies, but there are undoubtedly millions of us who don't even bother the doctor with our symptoms but self-medicate with over-the-counter remedies and/or experiment with changes in our diets. The UK charity Core found in a survey[1] that as many as 41 per cent of patients with digestive complaints had never visited their doctor to discuss their symptoms. Figures from the NHS for 2014 reveal that whilst there were over 18 million laxative products prescribed for constipation in general practice alone – a 35.5 per cent rise in 10 years – another 15.8 million laxative products were sold over the counter in pharmacies, at a cost of £58 million. Constipation also accounted for 666,287 hospital admissions in 2014.

Although some people may be perfectly capable of managing their own symptoms, believing them to be not serious enough or too embarrassing to tell their doctor about, there is an obvious danger that a more serious underlying condition might be missed, or that they may suffer in silence quite unnecessarily for years when often there is a simple solution that can resolve their symptoms.

IBS

Irritable bowel syndrome (IBS) is an umbrella term for a collection of abnormal bowel symptoms which can include constipation and/or diarrhoea, abdominal pain and bloating (see Chapter 3). IBS is estimated to affect as many as **nine million people**[2] (15 per cent of the population in the UK) at any one time.

IBS is embarrassing, debilitating, inconvenient and painful and has a massive impact on quality of life. Treating it costs the UK's NHS £1.2 billion a year. There's no cure, but there are a number of effective treatment options which can reduce the impact of the symptoms – if patients can get access to the right advice. Unfortunately, though, there's not a one-size-fits-all treatment for IBS; for instance, although eating more fibre can help people whose main IBS symptom is constipation it may *worsen* symptoms in patients who have diarrhoea as their main symptom (a condition known as IBS-D), and may not even be helpful to those whose constipation is caused by slow transit in the gut (where food and waste don't move as quickly as they should through the gut – see Chapter 9, page 162). Sadly though, some people never consult a doctor and suffer in silence, putting up with daily symptoms that can affect their education, careers, close relationships and social lives.

Inflammatory bowel disease (IBD)

Gastroenterologists are reporting an increase in diagnoses for inflammatory bowel diseases (IBD)[3] – Crohn's disease and ulcerative colitis; diseases which causes inflammation and/or ulceration of the lining of the gut. Recent studies published by the the Unversity of Edinburgh[4] reported a 76 per cent increase in incidence amongst children in Scotland since 1995. Across Europe the increase has been around 15 per cent over the same period. Doctors have various theories about why this is happening – one is that it's due to changes in diet and gut flora (known as the gut microbiome).

Coeliac disease, NCGS and the gluten-free trend

Blaming gluten (proteins found in wheat, barley and oats) for bloating and diarrhoea is currently very fashionable with sales of gluten-free foods such as bread, pasta and biscuits booming. In coeliac disease (see Chapter 4), the body's immune system mounts an inflammatory response to these foods, causing damage to the lining of the small bowel, disrupting the body's ability to absorb nutrients from food. Symptoms range from bloating and abdominal pain to diarrhoea and weight fluctuations. Coeliac disease can be diagnosed via a blood test and confirmed with an endoscopy and gut biopsy (see Glossary, page 180). Avoiding foods containing gluten causes the symptoms to disappear.

Research published by the University of Nottingham in 2014[5] found that although there has been a four-fold increase in the number of people diagnosed with coeliac disease over the past 20 years, three-quarters of cases – an estimated 500,000 people – remain undiagnosed. Meanwhile, although coeliac disease is estimated to affect only 1 per cent of the population, studies from New Zealand have shown that five times as many people are buying gluten-free foods than have been diagnosed as coeliac. Latest US figures[6] show that sales of gluten-free foods were estimated to reach $8.8 billion in 2014, an increase of 63 per cent from 2012–14.

So, if these people don't have coeliac disease what do they have then? Gluten-free products are usually at least 15 per cent more expensive than equivalent foods containing gluten – so presumably these consumers are sufficiently concerned (and in some cases desperate) that they are prepared to pay significantly more for their daily staples. Gastroenterologists have been puzzled for years by patients who swear blind they suffer bloating, pain and diarrhoea after they eat foods containing gluten but who test negative for coeliac disease. Increasingly, experts, are recognising another condition called non-coeliac gluten sensitivity (NCGS) – see Chapter 4 – which has similar symptoms to coeliac disease but without any of the markers or abnormalities that are found with coeliac disease when a blood test or gut biopsy is done. Dr Kamran Rostami, a gastroenterologist practising in Milton Keynes, wrote an article in the *British Medical Journal*[7] estimating that between four and seven million people may have this condition. Patients with NCGS who avoid gluten in their diet report their symptoms disappear, but experts say it's crucial they should be tested for coeliac disease while on a diet containing gluten, so coeliac disease can be eliminated first.

FODMAPs

Research carried out by the University of Monash in Australia[8] has established that 74 per cent of patients with IBS-type symptoms find their symptoms improve if they follow a diet of foods low in short-chained carbohydrates called FODMAPs (stands for fermentable oligo-, di-, monosaccharides and polyols) that are poorly absorbed in the bowel. Foods low in FODMAPs have been shown to reduce bloating, and diarrhoea symptoms. Foods high in FODMAPs include onions, garlic, beetroot, Savoy cabbage, apples, pears, mangos, fruit juices, beans and lentils, bread, pasta and in susceptible individuals, milk and dairy products. The catch is that a low FODMAP diet can be difficult to stick to. (For more on this, see Chapter 3, page 37.)

Bile acid diarrhoea

Another lesser known but common cause of diarrhoea is a condition called bile acid diarrhoea (BAD), which some experts believe is present in up to a third of the 3 million people in the UK who have been diagnosed with IBS with diarrhoea (IBS-D) as the predominant symptom. Never heard of it? Neither have most people, but BAD has features which set it apart from IBS (see Chapter 5). Symptoms can include up to 10 watery bowel movements a day, often with an urgent need to go and sometimes embarrassing faecal incontinence. There is also some bloating and abdominal pain.

The symptoms are caused by overproduction of bile acids in the liver and excess bile passing into the colon, causing watery diarrhoea. The condition can be diagnosed with a SeHCAT test comprising of two body scans (see Glossary). BAD can be treated with drugs including colestyramine which relieves the diarrhoea by binding to the unabsorbed bile acids, having a massive effect on quality of life.

Food allergies and intolerances

The incidence of food allergies and intolerances is on the increase,[9] particularly amongst children, and it's also becoming much more common to have multiple allergies.

Apart from food allergies, there appears to be an increasing recognition of lactose intolerance (a sugar found in cow's milk and sheep's milk and in other dairy products). This is *not* an allergy but an inability to digest lactose because of a deficiency in an enzyme called lactase. Lactose that has not been properly digested can produce diarrhoea, bloating and pain. People from many parts of the world have low lactase levels. In the UK, as many as one in five people are now believed to be lactose intolerant.[9,10]

Lactose intolerance can also develop as a temporary problem due to gut damage from undiagnosed coeliac disease. In most cases people who suffer this type of lactose intolerance will eventually be able to eat dairy products again if they follow a gluten-free diet, but it can take many months, or sometime years, for the gut to heal.

Cancer

Bowel cancer

Bowel cancer is overall the fourth most common cancer in the UK with breast or prostate cancer coming top followed by lung cancer. In the UK 41,600 people a year are diagnosed with the condition. Bowel cancer rates have risen by 14 per cent since the late 1970s.[11] Symptoms include changes in bowel movements and bleeding in the faeces, as well as unexplained weight loss. The strongest risk factor for bowel cancer is age though, as 80 per cent of cases occur in people aged 60 or over.[12] If you have a family history of bowel cancer at a young age be sure you have had the familial risk in your case explained (see Chapter 7).

Stomach, oesophageal and pancreatic cancers

People with chronic indigestion often wonder if they have cancer. To put the risk in perspective, the vast majority of people with indigestion-type symptoms will not develop cancer and the symptoms are related to cancer in only about 1 in 50 cases[13] – see Chapter 7, page 117.

- Stomach cancer is rare (around 6,000 cases a year in the UK) and is declining in the UK, with a 62 per cent drop in cases since the late 1970s,[14] but can cause gastric symptoms including acidity and burping, as well as feeling full, vomiting and weight loss.

- Difficulty swallowing with a sensation of food sticking in the chest could be a symptom of oesophageal cancer.

- Pancreatic cancer can cause pain and weight loss and often leads to jaundice.

Endoscopies, perhaps with blood or stool tests and ultrasound and other scans, will be able to exclude cancer quickly – usually within a couple of weeks.

Pelvic radiation disease (PRD)

Some cancer treatments such as radiotherapy to the pelvic area can also result in severe and frequent diarrhoea symptoms and can leave some patients housebound. This is known as pelvic radiation disease (see Chapter 7) and can start immediately after treatment or months or years later, so patients sometimes don't connect their symptoms with the cancer treatment. Experts estimate PRD affects around 17,000 new patients a year in the UK – more than the number of new patients with inflammatory bowel diseases – yet few people have heard of the condition.

Age, hormones and drug side effects

It is important to remember that there are a number of general issues to consider when you are assessing your own symptoms and what might be causing them.

- **Age.** Your gut function slows down as you get older making you more prone to constipation – due to a combination of less activity and reduced fluid and fibre intake and multiple drug side effects. Some studies[15] have found the prevalence of constipation is between 15 to 20 per cent in older people living at home and as high as 50 per cent for those living in nursing homes. Constipation sounds mildly inconvenient but can be painful and make people feel quite unwell, leading to associated problems such as haemorrhoids (piles) from straining and yet can be prevented and treated.

- **Hormones.** According to population studies twice as many women as men are affected by IBS. Many women with IBS report their symptoms flare up just before and during their menstrual periods, suggesting a role of sex hormones in the condition.[16] Fluctuating levels of the female sex hormone oestrogen may have a role. Similarly, 38 per cent of post-menopausal women also report altered gut function compared to 14 per cent of peri-menopausal women in one study.[17] Constipation is also a common problem in pregnant women, mainly because pregnancy homones slow down intestinal movements. The hormone progesterone relaxes muscles including the outside wall of the bowel.[18]

- **Drug side effects.** Some commonly prescribed drugs are well known for causing gut symptoms, including constipation and diarrhoea. Drugs sometimes associated with constipation include, antidepressants, certain painkillers, antiepileptics, antipsychotics, calcium supplements, diuretics and iron supplements.[19] Antibiotics, the gout drug allopurinol, digoxin, colchicine, cytotoxic drugs, antacids containing magnesium, the diabetes drug metformin, non-steroidal anti-inflammatory painkillers (such as ibuprofen), proton pump inhibitors (PPIs), selective serotonin reuptake inhibitors (SSRI antidepressants), statins, theophylline, thyroxine and high-dose vitamin C may all cause diarrhoea symptoms.[20]

Why are our guts playing up?

Scientists don't fully understand why the human race is currently suffering so much with gut issues, but the changes in diet and lifestyle we have seen in the last 150 years or so are unprecedented in human history. Here are some of the theories.

- **The hygiene hypothesis.** We've never been so clean – these days, in Western countries at least, daily washing is the norm, children play inside in centrally-heated, carpeted homes and not outside in the dirt, and their immune systems are not exposed to as many challenges from bacteria as in the past.

They're also less likely to share a room with a sibling and more likely to be a member of a smaller family, all factors which reduce exposure to pathogens while the immune system is developing. The theory is that these environmental differences are leading to changes in the bacteria which make up our gut flora and may be why certain diseases such as atopic allergies and gut disorders are on the increase.

- **Changes in diet.** Eating wheat is quite new for humans in evolutionary terms. Humans have existed for two million years but grains were first introduced in our diet only 10,000 years ago – so it may be that our guts are having trouble making the adjustments to eating these carbohydrates. Drinking milk as adults is even more recent and is linked to evolutionary changes in Europe. There have also been big changes in the way we cook and eat – relying more heavily on processed foods laden with fat, sugar and salt, takeaways and grazing on snacks between meals.

- **Gut flora.** Our bodies are 90 per cent bugs and only 10 per cent human tissue. Most bacteria live in the bowel, and there are 1,000 different organisms in symbiotic relationships (living together interdependently). Scientists now refer to this as the gut 'microbiome', an ecological system of microorganisms that exists within the gut. Over the last 50 years or so the way we live and our general environment have changed dramatically and so has our gut flora. This is likely to have had a significant effect on the way our immune systems are primed, argue some scientists, and an individual's gut bacteria may – it is proposed – play a role in whether they will develop certain illnesses or be obese or lean. Scientists have already identified types of bacteria that are associated with lean body weight and used it in transplants in mice. A US study published in late 2014 showed reductions in weight gain in the transplant mice and altered gut microbiome.[21]

- **Bottle-feeding and caesarean section deliveries.** Breastfeeding and vaginal deliveries are also associated with a lower rate of allergies in later life than children who are bottle-fed formula milk and delivered by caesarean section. Breast milk contains prebiotics which encourage the growth of beneficial gut flora, and vaginal deliveries expose babies to their mother's bowel bacteria which then colonise the baby's gut, giving them more protection.

- **Stresses of modern life.** We've never been busier with many of us cramming in long working days with commuting, child care and socialising. As the gut has some strong links with the brain and nervous systems, experts argue that stress may also trigger bowel symptoms in susceptible individuals.

Understanding your gut

As you read through this book it will be helpful if you have a general understanding of what the gut looks like and how the different parts fit together – see Figure 1.1. The gastrointestinal digestive tract is a muscular tube which is more than 30 feet long in total. It runs from the mouth to the oesophagus or gullet, through to the stomach and small intestine, on to the large intestine containing the colon and finally down to the rectum and anus. It moves food through the body via a series of muscular contractions (called peristalsis) before expelling waste and is dependent on the gall bladder (to store bile) and the liver (to eliminate toxins and produce digestive enzymes). The gut has its own nervous system (the enteric nervous system) and more nerves than the spinal cord, and is in constant dialogue with the brain via the vagus nerve.

The whole process from eating food to excreting waste takes on average 53 hours,[22] although this can vary considerably according to your diet, age and sex. With so many processes to go through it's perhaps not surprising that things can sometimes go wrong along the way.

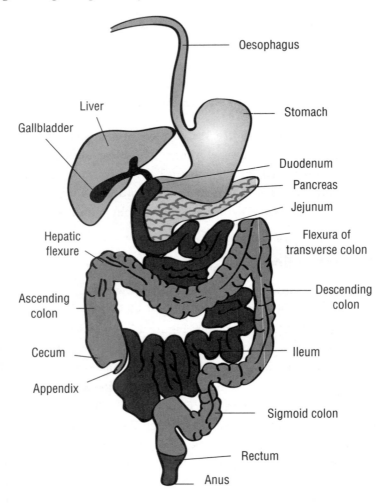

Figure 1.1 The digestive system

Ten fast facts about the gut

1. **Your gut contains 100 million neurons, more than in the spinal cord.** That churning feeling in your guts when you've got a job interview or presentation to make? It's not a coincidence and is a physical expression of your anxiety.

2. **The gut has its own nervous system known as the 'second brain'** as it can operate independently without instructions from the brain.

3. **The small intestine measures 22 feet (7 metres) in length** and its surface area would fill a 2,700 square feet (250 square metres) tennis court if laid out. It has a large surface area because it is lined with folds containing villi (finger-like projections) and micro villi which absorb food.

4. **The gut contains 100 trillion bacteria** and these outnumber human cells in the body by 10 to one – so actually we are more bacterial than human. Only 10 per cent of our DNA is Homo sapien – the vast majority is bacteria.

5. **Flatulence (or farting)** is a combination of swallowed air and gases produced by fermented bacteria in the gut. The rotten egg smell usally comes from hydrogen sulphide. The worst 'farty food' culprits are beans, pulses and lentils but also include fatty foods. Smelly wind is associated with garlic, onions and herbs belonging to the asafoetida family. Beer, white wine and fruit juice can produce smelly hydrogen sulphide farts in some people. On average we fart 15 times a day but up to 40 times a day is considered within a normal range.

6. **You don't need gravity to digest food** – the gut moves food down from the mouth towards the anus

by contracting the outer muscles of the gut – a bit like squeezing toothpaste. This is called peristalsis.

7. **Your stomach 'rumbles' all the time** – it's just that you can only hear it when it's empty as there is nothing to muffle the sound. The noise is caused by peristalsis (see above).

8. **It takes an average of 53 hours for food to make the journey from eating to excretion** – although like most things this can vary according to age, sex and type of diet.

9. **You can inherit your gut bacteria** – scientists have identified a type of bacteria called *Christensenella* which is associated with lean body mass. Transplanting it into mice reduced their body weight, so in the future this may be possible in humans too and help reduce obesity and obesity-related illnesses.

10. **At least 40 per cent of the population have at least one digestive symptom at any one time.**[23] The big four symptoms are abdominal pain, changes in bowel habit (constipation/diarrhoea), heartburn and indigestion.

Taking action

If you regularly feel uncomfortable after eating certain foods and notice your stomach becoming painful and swollen, or find you have daily diarrhoea, raging and repeated heartburn, or are struggling to pass stools due to constipation or cope with embarrassing flatulence – the good news is that you can do much to alleviate these symptoms and even stop them completely.

The key is finding out the cause and getting effective treatment – this may mean making dietary and lifestyle changes, trying drug treatments, psychological therapies, and in some cases undergoing surgery. We hope this book will help you unlock the secrets of what is up with your gut.

Chapter 2

How to use this book

- Red flag symptoms you shouldn't ignore
- Self-help tips for managing your symptoms
- Diagnostic tests

Before we launch into a more in-depth look at some of the gut complaints we've mentioned in Chapter 1, we thought it best to give you a gentle steer on how to make the best use of this book.

First of all, we see the book as complementing your medical care and advice, rather than replacing it – so always see your GP about symptoms that are troubling you. Your doctor will listen and take a full history of your symptoms and build up a complete picture of what is happening in your gut using his or her clinical judgement, and either order tests or refer you on to a specialist for further investigations.

We'd urge you not to self-medicate for the long term and always try to get a diagnosis for your gut complaints, as they are generally eminently treatable once correctly identified.

There is obviously a lot of overlap in gut symptoms – bleeding when you pass a stool is most likely going to be caused by piles (haemorrhoids), but in a small number of cases it could be a symptom of bowel cancer. This is where your doctor comes in – reading about the symptoms of different conditions will give you some useful pointers – but only a doctor can diagnose them.

Recognising red flags

However, there are some gut symptoms you should never ignore and we thought it best to flag them up here before going any further.

New *symptoms*

A lot of people endure symptoms such as pain, alternating bowel habits and food intolerance. These may have gone on for a long time, fluctuating in intensity and are sometimes helped by one or two dietary changes, and sometimes not. But recent changes are likely to be more serious than something that has persisted for years. If you had similar problems in your 20s to those in your 50s (and in between), it is unfortunate that you may have had to wait so long to get any answers, but it is not likely to be a life-threatening condition. If the symptoms have just started, it is far more worrying. Don't be embarrassed. Help your GP assess what needs to be done. Be sure to describe how long you have had the symptoms and explain exactly what you mean.

In particular, be sure to tell your GP about the following symptoms as they may indicate a serious condition:
- abdominal pain and fever
- anaemia
- blood in your stools
- change in bowel habits
- jaundice and definite lumps you can feel
- unexplained weight loss.

Abdominal pain and fever

Fever and sharp, stabbing abdominal pain can have several causes and you may need to go to A&E or even call an ambulance if these are severe and sudden in onset.

Anaemia

Anaemia, which will make you look pale and feel tired, may be due to hidden ('occult') blood loss, and your GP may organise for you to have an endoscopy and/or colonoscopy (see Glossary, page 181), together with blood tests for coeliac disease, iron, B12 and folate deficiency.

Blood in your stools

Blood in your stools must be investigated. If it occurs only on wiping the anus with toilet tissue, it may just be haemorrhoids (piles) or an anal fissure (tear), but this should be checked by an examination, and then perhaps by a limited flexible sigmoidoscopy (see Glossary, page 183). If there is blood mixed in with the stools, you should be referred to a gastroenterologist or colorectal surgeon and have further tests, such as colonoscopy (or possibly a CT scan – see Glossary, page 181), to be certain bowel cancer and ulcerative colitis have been excluded. These are major diseases which are much more successfully treated if caught early and are not difficult to diagnose with the proper tests, so get your GP to refer you to a gastroenterologist if you suspect one of these.

Although bowel cancer increases in likelihood as you get older, it is common enough that people aged 40 to 50 or younger can get it. If you know that you have a family history of bowel cancer you are also more at risk. The good news is that, when you have had a colonoscopy, you can be sure for quite a long time (several years) that this has been excluded as the cause of your symptoms. The faecal calprotectin test (see Glossary, page 183) is now also useful in predicting if you do need a colonoscopy. If you are older, be sure to get the routine screening tests that are now offered.

Change in bowel habits

If you have a recent change in your bowel habit, then tell your GP and be prepared to get more tests. Clearly, if everyone in your family has just got the same symptoms after eating the same food, or you have just come back from an area where gastroenteritis is common, and the symptoms are not too bad, you can wait a week or two to see whether things go back to normal. But if they do not, and particularly if there is blood in the stools, then you **MUST** get tests.

Jaundice and definite lumps you can feel

Jaundice symptoms (yellow eyes and skin) and definite lumps, particularly if they are tender, must not be ignored. The lumps may turn out to be only hard faeces but you want to be sure that a definite diagnosis is made in case it might be an inflamed gall bladder, an ovarian or another cyst, or possibly a stomach or bowel tumour. Hernias in the groin or in other places in the abdomen may also feel like painful lumps and can also cause problems until they are treated.

Unexplained weight loss

Unexplained weight loss is important and will lead to other blood tests and probably hospital referral. Sometimes there is a gut disease (coeliac disease or Crohn's disease, for instance) or cancer, but in other cases can be due to an endocrine disorder, such as an over-active thyroid, or to a wide range of other disorders, including neurological or mental health problems (you cannot buy, cook or chew your food), or cannot easily eat (dental problems, for instance or Alzheimer's). These should be fairly easy for your GP to diagnose.

Working out what's wrong

So, apart from the red flag symptoms listed above, where do you start when trying to work out what's up with your gut?

You can help yourself and your doctor by:

- **Keeping a diary of your symptoms.** It helps your doctor make a diagnosis if you can be specific about how long you've had your symptoms, what they are, what seems to trigger them or whether they are present all the time, and how much weight you have lost. Keeping a diary of your gut symptoms will help you remember and give your doctor valuable information. One gastroenterologist has told us how increasingly patients will photograph or video their bloated stomachs on their mobile phones to document their symptoms.

- **Not being embarrassed.** People literally die of embarrassment because they can't get their heads round describing their stools/piles/diarrhoea to their doctors. Get over it. If you don't like describing what your poo looks like ask your doctor if you can point it out on the Bristol Stool Chart (see Figure 9.1, page 178).

- **Mentioning any family history of gut disease to your doctor.** Some complaints do have a genetic basis so it will be another piece in the jigsaw for your doctor if you can supply details of conditions such as bowel cancer or inflammatory bowel diseases in your immediate family. (Volunteer this if they don't ask you first.)

- **Not cutting out food groups on a hunch.** If you do have an autoimmune condition, such as coeliac disease, where the body reacts to gluten and causes bowel symptoms, it's important you don't cut out any foods you suspect are to blame, such as bread or breakfast cereals, until your condition has been fully investigated. This is because you may need a gut biopsy to confirm your diagnosis (the villi – finger-like projections in the gut which absorb nutrients – will be damaged and shrunken if you have coeliac disease) and if you have stopped eating gluten they may have returned to normal, giving a false negative diagnosis.

- **Being persistent.** If your doctor has told you to eat more bran to help with constipation and your symptoms are getting worse, go back and tell him or her. Whilst eating more fibre helps in a lot of cases of constipation, in up to 30 per cent of cases it doesn't. (The cause could be slow transit in the gut (see Chapter 9, page 162), in which case too much fibre will make it worse!)

- **Not self-medicating for the long term.** Obviously it's fine to buy over-the-counter remedies if your gut problems are short term, but if you are relying on laxatives, antacids or anti-diarrhoea medication in the long term it's advisable to see a doctor and find out the underlying cause.

- **Finding reliable sources of information.** There are an awful lot of 'snake oil' salesmen out there on the internet, peddling dodgy cures or extreme diets with no good science to recommend them. Charities are good sources of accurate information about managing your condition and their online resources are written in a reader-friendly consumer style. Don't forget organisations such as NICE (the National Institute for Health and Care Excellence) produce guideline summaries on the management of health conditions written especially for patients, setting out clearly what investigations and treatments are recommended.

Tests and investigations

If your doctor suspects certain gut conditions you may need to have a number of blood tests, investigations and scans to confirm/eliminate a diagnosis. Table 2.1 summarises how the major gut problems may be tested for, the detail of which is explained later in the book and in the Glossary.

Table 2.1 Diagnosing key gut diseases

Condition	Tests
Bowel cancer	Colonoscopy (and biopsy) / CT scan
Ulcerative colitis/ Crohn's disease	Biopsies from colonoscopy/sigmoidoscopy. CT scan/MRI (and blood and faecal tests)
Coeliac (allergy to gluten)	Blood test and gut biopsies
Anaemia	Endoscopies are accurate for identifying sources of loss of blood. Blood testing for coeliac disease will be done in case this is the cause of ongoing loss of blood
Peptic ulcers	The bacterium *Helicobacter pylori* is the main cause; there is a stool test, or sometimes a breath test, that can be done to see if it is present
Gallstones	Ultrasound will diagnose these easily and may pick up some other liver problems

The chapters that follow describe gut symptoms in more detail, give the background of the latest thinking on the causes of gut diseases and advise on the best treatments currently available. We hope they'll help you find the answers to what's up with your gut.

Chapter 3

Irritable bowel syndrome (IBS)

Symptom checker

- Diarrhoea
- Bloating
- Constipation
- Pain in the rectum
- Urgency to pass stools
- Abdominal cramps and spasms often relieved by going to the loo

---

Could you have IBS?

Chances are that if you've suffered from persistent bloating, stomach pain and diarrhoea/constipation for long enough the words irritable bowel syndrome (IBS) will have been mentioned to you (or you will have figured it out yourself).

IBS is a medical term used by doctors to describe a collection of gut symptoms – you might have some or all of them. IBS is estimated to affect as many as one in four of us at some point in our lives and one in 10 of those affected have symptoms severe enough to see a doctor about.

Globally IBS is estimated to affect 5 to 11 per cent of the population, peaking in the third and fourth decades of life and more commonly affecting women.[1] Estimates in the UK vary but current thinking is that IBS may affect around 15 per cent of the population (nine million people) (see IBS Network). Experts have described IBS as a 'chronic, relapsing and life-long' disorder.[2]

Although there's a perception that IBS is something relatively minor (perhaps because it won't kill you and because lots of people have it to some degree), nevertheless it can be extremely debilitating, painful, inconvenient and embarrassing and has a huge impact on quality of life.[3] If you have uncontrolled IBS you may underperform at school, have to take time off work, have relationship problems and even stop going out because the symptoms can have such an impact and be socially embarrassing. Some people end up housebound because they are so terrified of having some sort of accident.

And there's no cure for IBS – so managing your symptoms is often a case of trial and error (albeit under expert medical supervision, although often that's not the case, unfortunately) and trying different dietary and lifestyle changes and/or medications or psychological therapies.

What are the symptoms?

Apart from diarrhoea and/or constipation, symptoms can include bloating and swelling of the abdomen, abdominal pain, cramps and spasms, often relieved by going to the loo. Other symptoms may include an urgent need to dash to the toilet, a sharp pain inside the rectum and sensation of incomplete bowel movement, flatulence and wind, mucus in stools and/or indigestion/heartburn. In a minority of cases IBS may involve bowel incontinence, or pain during sex – it can be grim and extremely hard to live with.[4]

Symptoms can also occur in other parts of the body. These symptoms may include headache, dizziness, backache, passing urine more frequently, muscle and joint pain, belching, nausea, anxiety, depression, fatigue and tiredness.[5]

Most people will suffer from attacks of symptoms that gradually die down and then recur. You may notice that certain foods trigger symptoms which last a few days or that stress and anxiety, work pressures, exam worries, money difficulties, divorce or bereavement may precede and coincide with your symptoms starting. In women, IBS symptoms often flare just before or at the start of a menstrual period.

A minority of IBS sufferers are more unfortunate and suffer persistent severe symptoms that never go away.

You wouldn't get an IBS diagnosis until typically you had been suffering from symptoms for at least six months.[6]

How is IBS diagnosed?

There are lots of difficulties surrounding making an IBS diagnosis. The first is that each IBS symptom can also be a sign of other gut disorders, and your doctor will use his/her skills in taking a medical history to decide whether tests and investigations are needed to eliminate these (see Box 3.1 below). The obvious ones are infections (everyone has had food poisoning or gastroenteritis lasting a few days at some point); but others include cancers of the digestive tract and ovaries; coeliac disease, where symptoms are triggered by gluten in barley, wheat and rye; and inflammatory bowel diseases, including Crohn's disease and ulcerative colitis.

Less well known diseases which may cause some IBS-type symptoms include non-coeliac gluten-sensitivity (page 72), bile acid diarrhoea (page 79) and 'SIBO' (page 90).

Diagnosis is made by identifying a typical pattern of symptoms and the absence of any 'red flag' symptoms (see Chapter 2) that may indicate structural diseases of the bowel, so it's partly a process of elimination. These red flags include unexplained weight loss, bleeding in the faeces or from the back passage and new bowel symptoms in people aged over 50 – e.g. diarrhoea or constipation for the first time – or a family history of bowel or ovarian cancer.

Is there a test for IBS?

IBS is a disorder of gut function or how the gut works – the gut itself doesn't become damaged – so there is nothing you can easily test for or spot in a biopsy. When X-rays and endoscopies (see Glossary, page 181) and other diagnostic tests are carried out in IBS patients the results do not reveal any obvious structural problems. Similarly, blood and stool tests are normal. Unfortunately, as yet there are no tests that can reveal a biomarker for IBS either (although some possibilities have recently been identified).

In the past people with IBS say they been unfairly labelled as hypochondriacs or told their symptoms were 'psychosomatic', but gastroenterologists today do agree that even if some of the symptoms of IBS may be triggered by stress or anxiety, they are still very real physical symptoms and by no means imaginary or 'all in the mind'. Specialised tests can show changes in the motility of the gut or detect hypersensitivity with greater awareness of sensation.

It is really helpful for your GP if you can keep a diary of your symptoms so that you are able to describe in detail their severity and frequency.

Box 3.1 NICE Guidelines on IBS

The UK's National Institute for Health and Care Excellence (NICE) guideline on diagnosis and treatment of IBS from 2008, as updated in 2015,[7] says all patients presenting with IBS symptoms should be assessed and examined for anaemia, abdominal and rectal masses and inflammatory markers for inflammatory bowel diseases. Women with symptoms suggestive of ovarian cancer should be offered blood screening tests for serum CA125, a biomarker for ovarian cancer.

The guideline goes on to state:

1.1.1.1 Healthcare professionals should consider assessment for IBS if the person reports having had any of the following symptoms for at least 6 months:
- Abdominal pain or discomfort
- Bloating
- Change in bowel habit. [2008]

1.1.1.2 All people presenting with possible IBS symptoms should be asked if they have any of the following 'red flag' indicators and should be referred to secondary care for further investigation if any are present:[4]
- unintentional and unexplained weight loss
- rectal bleeding
- a family history of bowel or ovarian cancer
- a change in bowel habit to looser and/or more frequent stools persisting for more than six weeks in a person aged over 60 years. [2008]

1.1.1.3 All people presenting with possible IBS symptoms should be assessed and clinically examined for the following 'red flag' indicators and should be referred to secondary care for further investigation if any are present:

- anaemia
- abdominal masses
- rectal masses
- inflammatory markers for inflammatory bowel disease.

Measure serum CA125 in primary care in women with symptoms that suggest ovarian cancer in line with the NICE guideline on ovarian cancer.[8] [2008]

1.1.1.4 A diagnosis of IBS should be considered only if the person has abdominal pain or discomfort that is either relieved by defaecation or associated with altered bowel frequency or stool form. This should be accompanied by at least two of the following four symptoms:

- altered stool passage (straining, urgency, incomplete evacuation)
- abdominal bloating (more common in women than men), distension, tension or hardness
- symptoms made worse by eating
- passage of mucus.

Other features such as lethargy, nausea, backache and bladder symptoms are common in people with IBS, and may be used to support the diagnosis. [2008]

What tests can you expect? NICE recommends that people who meet the above diagnostic criteria should then be investigated with a full blood count, a blood test for erythrocyte sedimentation or plasma viscosity, a C-reactive protein (all measures of inflammation in the body) and antibody testing for coeliac disease.

Source: NICE [2008, updated 2015].[8] Reproduced with permission.

Whilst in some cases you may think you can manage your IBS symptoms without seeing your GP, it makes better sense to get a confirmed diagnosis as your symptoms just might have a more serious underlying cause, such as coeliac disease (see Chapter 4, page 57 – an estimated three-quarters of all coeliacs remain undiagnosed in the UK), inflammatory bowel disease (Chapter 6, page 95), ulcers (Chapter 8, page 148) or cancer (Chapter 7, page 117), which a doctor may be able to pick up on. Even if you are confirmed as having IBS, a doctor can also advise you on the full range of treatments available and if need be refer you on to a specialist and/or dietitian.

Who gets IBS?

IBS is extremely common in Western countries. Estimates vary but prevalence in England and Wales is estimated at between 10 and 20 per cent. Likewise in the US, IBS is estimated to affect 30 million people, making it the most common gastrointestinal disorder.

Symptoms are common in the 20 to 30 year age group but can affect all age groups, including children and teenagers and also the elderly. One US study found 14 per cent of high school students and 6 per cent of middle school students had IBS. It is also twice as common in women as it is in men. In the UK around

13 per cent of women and 5 per cent of men are reported to have IBS, for instance.[9]

What causes IBS?

So what causes IBS? Is it your genes, food that you eat, stress, hormones, anxiety and other psychological problems or even an infection or changes in your gut bacteria (known as the gut microbiome) or a combination of some of these factors?

The short answer is that nobody knows for sure, although there's likely to be different causes for specific symptoms such as diarrhoea, pain or bloating. Here's a summary of some of the very latest thinking.

Genetic and environmental triggers

IBS symptoms can coincide with busy and/or stressful periods in life – becoming a parent, important exams, divorce, money worries, putting in long hours at work, unemployment – all seem to take their toll and trigger symptoms – although obviously not in everyone.

The thinking is that some individuals are more susceptible to IBS than others, probably through their genetic makeup – but as yet no specific genes have been identified. One study published in 2014 by scientists at the Technische Universtaet Muenchen (TUM)[10] did identify that one group of IBS patients had a gene mutation of the SCN5A gene. They found the defect affected a sodium channel in the smooth muscles of the GI tract – so this is another area where scientific understanding is advancing.

Psychological issues

IBS is also reported to be more common in people who suffer from stress, anxiety and depression and those suffering from post-traumatic stress disorder.[11] IBS patients are also more likely to have suffered a trauma or a number of big stressful life events such as divorce, bereavement or abuse. This comes as no surprise though, as scientists know that the gut has its own nervous system which operates completely independently from the brain – the enteric nervous system, a network of neurons (nerve cells) that govern the function of the gastrointestinal system. As mentioned in Chapter 1, it has even been referred to by neuro-gastroenterologists as 'the second brain'.

Experts also argue that having IBS symptoms might induce psychological symptoms and it's difficult to establish which comes first in a chicken-and-egg-type scenario. Also some IBS sufferers have no symptoms of anxiety and stress. To confuse matters further, there's also a condition called non-coeliac gluten sensitivity (see page 72).

Infections and gut microbiota

Some research has also suggested that IBS can be triggered by a severe gastric infection, such as gastroenteritis in certain susceptible individuals. After a severe outbreak of waterborne dysentery was reported in Walkerton, Ontario, in Canada, for instance, up to a third of those who caught an infection from an infected water supply went onto to develop persistent symptoms of IBS, even though no ongoing infection was detected.[12] Another study found that one in four cases of patients who had been hospitalised for gastroenteritis reported their IBS symptoms started after the attack. Other studies have reported the incidence of post-infection IBS at between 7 and 33 per cent.[13]

Another study carried out by scientists at TUM's Department of Human Biology in Munich, Germany, demonstrated that micro-inflammation of the gut mucosa (the innermost lining of the gut which acts as a 'second skin' in the immune system) can cause sensitisation of the gut's enteric nervous system. One of the lead researchers said the irritated mucosa produced more neuroactive chemicals, such as serotonin and histamine, and suggested these could be the cause of unpleasant IBS symptoms. The researchers found that IBS symptoms improved when they were given antihistamines.[14]

Post-infection IBS after a bout of gastroenteritis is also one of the strongest indications for the importance of the gut microbiota. The human intestine is colonised by tens of millions of micro-organisms (collectively known as the gut microbiota) and these can be influenced by infection, diet, age and antibiotic treatment. Doctors have already discovered that changing the gut microbiota by giving probiotic supplements (live cultures of certain bacteria that normally inhabit the colon) can alleviate IBS symptoms such as bloating and diarrhoea in some cases[15] (see below, page 48).

Hormones

Hormones are thought to play a part in triggering IBS symptoms. Some women for instance report IBS symptoms are worse at the time of their menstrual periods with greater rectal sensitivity and looser stools.[16] Post- and peri-menopausal women also report more gastrointestinal symptoms, such as abdominal bloating. Thirty eight per cent of post-menopausal women in one study reported altered gut function in contrast to 14 per cent of pre-menopausal women. The prevalence of IBS-type symptoms peaked in the menopausal years between 40 and 49 to 36 per cent.[17]

Food and food sensitivities

Some people who have IBS symptoms are convinced their symptoms are triggered by particular foods, including caffeine, alcohol, fibre and fats – although scientists say the evidence is conflicting on some foods and lacking in others.

Whilst food allergies involving an immune response are the cause of IBS-type symptoms in less than 3 per cent of cases,[18] food intolerances where the body reacts to chemical components of food may trigger symptoms. Recent studies have shown that high numbers of people with IBS symptoms have a sensitivity to gluten (page 72). A 2015 study by Bijan Shahbazkhani et al concluded, 'a large number of patients labelled as IBS are senstitive to gluten'. However, experts believe an individual has in the first place to have a sensitive or intolerant gut that reacts to foods that stimulate or produce gas – so although foods may be the trigger for symptoms they are not the underlying cause.

Although food allergies usually produce immediate symptoms, including vomiting, diarrhoea and stomach pain, as well as swelling around the mouth and throat, headaches and rashes, sometimes the reaction is less obvious and delayed for several days so it can be more difficult to identify the cause. If you notice your gut reacts to certain foods then keep a careful food diary of your symptoms and seek medical advice. It's really important you don't attempt to self-diagnose and cut out certain foods groups without seeing a doctor first – a medical professional will be able to eliminate conditions such as coeliac disease (see Chapter 4, page 59) where the body has an adverse reaction to gluten (a protein found in wheat, barley and rye), with blood tests and sometimes gut biopsies. Coeliac disease affects around 1 per cent of the population and symptoms may include bloating, diarrhoea, stomach pain and fatigue and so can be confused with IBS. It's not a food intolerance, however, but an autoimmune condition where the body's immune system mistakes gluten as a threat and attacks it with antibodies, damaging the lining of the gut.

Milk intolerance

According to the charity Allergy UK, milk is the biggest cause of food intolerance in the UK, with stomach or abdominal discomfort, bloating and diarrhoea the most commonly reported symptoms.[19] Most people who experience gut problems after eating dairy products do not have an allergy to milk but an intolerance to lactose, a sugar found in milk, or to some of the proteins in milk. They lack an enzyme called lactase which digests lactose, so lactose is not broken down and passes on through the digestive system, causing wind, bloating and diarrhoea. If you or your ancestors have moved to the UK from China, Africa or the Caribbean there is a strong likelihood that your genetic makeup makes you more likely to be lactose intolerant. If your genetic heritage is from the Indian subcontinent, the Middle East or possibly some Mediterranean countries then it is still quite likely you could be lactose intolerant. Even in northern Europeans, the chances of being lactose intolerant can be as high as one in 10.

Research has shown that 44 per cent of people who describe themselves as dairy intolerant have self-diagnosed themselves and cut out all dairy products without ever being carefully tested. If this has worked for you then you have found out the cause of your problem. Be sure to replace dairy products with other sources of calcium such as sardines, dried fruit, soya milk or cereals fortified with calcium. However, if you do suspect you have lactose intolerance but are not sure, see your GP and ask for a glucose hydrogen breath test (see Glossary, page 183). If you are found to be lactose intolerant, the treatment is cutting out milk and dairy products.

Other food intolerances

The IBS Network charity advises that wheat, milk, some fruits, onions, leeks and garlic, beetroot, pulses (peas, beans and lentils), cereal husks, coffee, red meat, fried food, ready-meals rich in fat, chocolate, butter and cream, may all trigger IBS symptoms.

In the past people with IBS were advised to eat more fibre-rich foods and whilst this can be helpful in those who have constipation as their main symptom, too much fibre can actually make symptoms worse in people who have diarrhoea as their predominant symptom. Even in some people who suffer constipation, fibre may not be helpful (see page 162, slow-transit constipation).

The British Dietetics Association[20] recommends keeping a food and symptom diary to try and identify which foods may be to blame. For instance, lactose found in milk and dairy products can cause wind and bloating, and broccoli, sprouts, cabbage and cauliflower, and sugar-free mints containing sorbitol, can all produce gas.

FODMAPs

There is increasing interest in the role of FODMAPs (fermentable oligosaccharides, disaccharides, monosaccharides and polyols) in managing IBS symptoms – these are short-chain carbohydrates (sugars) or sugar alcohols that are found in a wide range of foods and drinks. FODMAPs are poorly absorbed in the small intestine and can enter the colon where they are fermented by bacteria, which stretches the sensitive bowel causing bloating, a swollen tummy, wind and diarrhoea. Most people with normal gut function and gut bacteria are able to digest FODMAPs, but in those with a sensitive gut and altered gut flora they can cause troublesome symptoms.

The first paper grouping these foods together and using the term FODMAPs was published in 2005[21] and has since generated intense interest and further research studies.[22] Foods high in FODMAPs include onions, garlic, beetroot, Savoy cabbage, apples, pears, mangos, and, in susceptible individuals, milk and dairy products. Bread also contains FODMAPs and when consumed as a staple may lead to significant symptoms. A number of studies have shown that following a low FODMAP diet can improve IBS symptoms in 74 per cent of cases – although it's by no means a cure.[23]

Six short-chained carbohydrates in particular have been identified as being problematic for people with sensitive guts – see Table 3.1.

Table 3.1 FODMAPS in foods

FODMAPS	Richest food sources
Fructo-oligosaccharides (fructan)	Wheat, rye, onions, garlic and artichokes
Galacto-oligosaccharides	Legumes
Lactose	Milk
Fructose	Honey, apples, pears, water, melon, mango
Sorbitol	Apples, pears, stone fruits, sugar-free mints and gum
Mannitol	Mushrooms, cauliflower, sugar-free mints and gum

Source: Barrett and Gibson, 2012.[23]

The candidiasis hypersensitivity theory

Some alternative health practitioners believe hypersensitivity to *Candida albicans* – a yeast that grows on the body (usually the skin) and normally causes no problems – may be to blame for IBS symptoms and a range of other unexplained issues. It has been put forward as an explanation for symptoms such as bloating , fatigue, diarrhoea, constipation, muscle and joint pain and cravings for sugar to name but a few. The theory – first put forward in the early

1980s – is that people with these problems suffer from an allergy to *Candida albicans*, but this has not been accepted as a medical diagnosis. The IBS Network sums it up nicely when it says, 'In a nutshell there's no credible scientific evidence to support the notion that candidiasis is a cause of IBS.'

There are plenty of books written about *Candida* hypersensitivity; the first was *The Yeast Connection* by Dr William Crook MD in 1983 who argued these symptoms often began when something upset the balance between yeast and so-called 'friendly' bacteria in the intestine. This disruption may follow a course of antibiotics or steroids, taking the contraceptive pill or damage to the lining of the stomach caused by non-steroidal anti- inflammatory drugs (NSAIDs) it has been argued.

Our view is that it is an interesting theory – but that's all. The 'treatments' advocated by alternative health practitioners include a restricted diet (cutting out foods containing yeast and sugar and then reintroducing them and reassessing), and anti-fungal treatments – but again, there's no scientific evidence that they work and critics point out that cutting out food groups for no good reason is not sensible and that antifungal treatments do have side effects. Yes, some patients do claim to feel better after following these diets, but the improvement could be due to the placebo effect or just eating a generally healthier diet which is lower in sugar and junk food. There is also the risk that believing your symptoms are due to *Candida* could stop you getting a diagnosis for what is really causing your symptoms – inflammatory bowel disease, for example.

Similarly, there is another related theory popular with alternative health practitioners called the 'leaky gut syndrome'. This idea is that the mucosal lining of the gut becomes damaged by poor diet, antibiotics and yeast overgrowth causing food, toxins and bacteria to 'leak' from inside the bowel into the bloodstream causing widespread symptoms. The hypothesis is that the particles which leak across into the bloodstream trigger an immune response causing inflammation all over the body – resulting in a range of symptoms including migraine, lupus, diabetes, eczema, autism, food allergies and chronic fatigue. Again, this not a medically recognised diagnosis, and we are merely mentioning it here in case you had come across it; we are not confirming that it exists.

For these reasons this book is sticking to medically recognised conditions and treatments.

Treatments for IBS

Unfortunately, at the moment there's no one cure or treatment that will help all IBS sufferers. But that doesn't mean it is a hopeless situation – far from it. There are many treatments that can help you manage your particular symptoms better and reduce their severity and frequency. Too many patients give up trying to find the triggers for their symptoms and resign themselves to living with what can be quite debilitating and restricting symptoms. One UK study found that people with IBS had much poorer general health status compared with the general population and one third had missed at least one day's work in the previous four weeks due to their symptoms.[24] They will always have an eye out for the nearest toilet and even turn down work opportunities or social invitations for fear of embarrassment.

Taking control of your own health and learning what triggers your symptoms can help you manage your IBS symptoms better. Whilst your GP can give you advice about changing your diet and lifestyle and managing stress better, as well as prescribing anti-spasmodic drugs to control diarrhoea and bulking agents to help prevent constipation, it really is only you who knows your own body.

If you enter a Google search for treatments for IBS 2.4 million hits appear, so it can be confusing and bewildering to try and find advice which is reliable and based on scientific studies. Here are some pointers to help you get your gut health back on track.

24 ways to manage your IBS

Managing your IBS relies on you getting to know your body and what foods and other environmental factors, such as stress, depression and alcohol, can affect your gut function.

1. See your doctor

Yes it sounds obvious – but so many people with IBS-type symptoms never bother to see a doctor and suffer unnecessarily or leave it too late with serious conditions such as colon cancer or ovarian cancer. Don't let this happen to you. Your doctor will be able to identify any red flag symptoms, such as bleeding from the back passage, unexplained weight loss, feeling too full after eating only small amounts and abdominal bloating, and order the appropriate investigations or specialist referrals to make the diagnoses early, when treatment will be simpler and more effective.

2. Keep a food and symptom diary

This is the easiest way to pinpoint which foods may be triggering your symptoms. Once you have identified them, try cutting them out of your diet and see what difference it makes. It really is best to do this under medical supervision so your doctor can eliminate any more serious underlying condition. Some IBS patients find that they may be able to tolerate the foods again if they are reintroduced slowly. If you are senstive to gluten though, it's important to get tested for coeliac disease before excluding it from your diet (page 65).

3. Go easy on fibre – especially bran

You may have picked up somewhere that high-fibre foods, such as bran, whole grains and fruits and vegetables, are healthy and good for you and that's generally true, especially if constipation is your main symptom (but if you do use fibre, increase it gradually). But doctors are no longer convinced that bran is always helpful. A 1994 study[26] carried out by Francis & Whorwell, for instance, found that in 55 of 100 consecutive IBS patients referred to secondary care (hospital), eating more bran made IBS symptoms worse. They found it caused abdominal disturbance, bloating and pain and also raised the possibility that excessive consumption of bran may actually be creating patients with IBS by exacerbating mild cases. When Whorwell and colleagues repeated the study in primary care (patients attending a GP surgery) in 2006, however, bran was found to improve symptoms in 27 per cent of cases and made symptoms worse in 22 per cent and made no difference in the remainder.[27] In 2008, the UK's National Institute for Health and Clinical Excellence[28] recommended that people with IBS should be discouraged from eating insoluble fibre, including bran. NICE recommended that if an increase in dietary fibre is required it should be soluble fibre, such as ispaghula powder or oats.

4. Find out about the low FODMAP diet

As we've already said above (page 37), foods high in FODMAPs, including certain fruits and vegetables, can also exacerbate symptoms. Many dietitians are now trained in the low FODMAP diet and can give you advice about how to eliminate and reintroduce foods high in these sugars, so ask your doctor for a referral. A low FODMAP diet has been found to reduce symptoms in around 74 per cent of cases and is now being suggested as a first-line treatment by some doctors. It's not a cure (and can be quite hard to stick to) but may dramatically reduce your symptoms and make them easier to live with. Latest updated guidance from NICE published in 2015 says that if a person's IBS persists while following general lifestyle and dietary advice, then single food avoidance and exclusion diets, such as the low FODMAP diet, may be recommended, but 'only under the guidance of a healthcare professional with expertise in dietary management'.[28]

5. Go easy on fatty foods

Processed foods tend to have a high fat content which can also trigger symptoms in IBS patients. Don't live on takeaways and ready meals, chocolate and crisps, and cook for yourself from scratch where possible, avoiding chips, pizzas and curries (particularly creamy sauces).

6. Think about what you're drinking as well as what you eat

Coffee, tea, cola, alcohol and orange juice are some of the drinks that IBS patients report can trigger symptoms. If you notice any symptoms try caffeine-free or herbal teas and coffees and drink water instead of orange juice. Aim to drink eight glasses (two litres) of fluid a day but limit caffeinated drinks to no more than three and orange juice to one glass.

7. Limit fresh fruit to three portions a day

This was NICE's recommendation for IBS sufferers in 2008 – presumably because of both the high fibre and FODMAP content. It's also said to be helpful to avoid the skin, pips and pith from fruit and vegetables, as these may be difficult to digest.

8. Eat porridge to stop wind

If you suffer from wind, try eating porridge or another oat-based cereal for breakfast and up to one tablespoon of linseeds a day – that's the recommendation from the National Institute for Health and Care Excellence.

9. Take enough time to eat

Experts recommend not eating on the hoof, not skipping meals and avoiding eating too close to bedtime, as all can affect digestion. Aim for three meals a day and don't rush your meals

– sit down at the table and enjoy them. Missing meals can mean that you're more likely to eat high-fat foods.

10. Get checked for lactose intolerance

Lactose is found in milk and dairy products, which is normally digested by an enzyme called lactase – however, as we've said earlier in the book (page 35), some people don't have enough of this. The main symptoms of lactose intolerance are flatulence, diarrhoea, bloating and stomach cramps, usually starting quite soon after you've eaten dairy products. Sometimes this happens after a stomach upset or another gut disease, including coeliac disease or inflammatory bowel disease – this type of lactose intolerance is called secondary lactose intolerance (there's another inherited type too) and is usually a temporary problem which will eventually clear. For others the symptoms last much longer. You can develop secondary lactose intolerance at any age but the most common time to develop symptoms is between the ages of 20 and 40. Switching to a lactose-free diet may greatly improve symptoms, but it can be difficult to eliminate lactose from your diet completely because lactose is used in so many processed foods, including chocolate, salad dressings, boiled sweets, instant soups, some breads and cereals, and processed cooked meats. Usually there is only a small amount of lactose in yoghurts and cheese. Alternatives to lactose products include milks and yoghurts made from soya, coconuts and almonds and foods labelled as lactose-free. Take care though that you don't miss out on the important nutrients in dairy foods, including calcium and vitamin D – both needed for strong bones. Eat calcium-rich foods, such as tinned pilchards, leafy green vegetables or dried fruit, to ensure you get enough calcium from your diet, or buy food fortified with calcium, such as fruit juices or breakfast cereals. You could also consider taking a calcium or vitamin D supplement. You can also buy lactase supplements to help with digestion of lactose and milk with added lactase.

11. Learn to relax

Stress, working too hard and anxiety don't cause IBS but can make IBS symptoms worse, affecting their onset, severity and duration. If you have too much stress in your life it's important you tackle the causes to try and reduce it – admittedly easier said than done in a lot of cases, but if you can at least learn how to handle it better with relaxation techniques your symptoms might ease. Try deep breathing exercises, winding down before bed in a warm bath or meditation techniques. Even a brisk walk in fresh air may help. The latest updated guidance from NICE published in February 2015 suggests a positive effect, but evidence is 'limited and insufficient to make any recommendations'.

12. Try prescription drug treatments

Standard treatments include:

- **Antispasmodics for cramps.** These include therapeutic peppermint oil and mebeverine and they work by relaxing muscles in the gut, relieving pain and cramping.

- **Laxatives.** Bulk-forming laxatives, such as Fybogel (ispaghula husk), help constipation by swelling as they absorb water, increasing bulk in the bowel, helping you have more regular bowel movements and absorb water and softening your stools. Another type of laxative is Movicol, which contains macrogol, polyethylene glycol and an inert substance that pass through the gut.

- **Antimotility medicines.** These are usually recommended for IBS-related diarrhoea, and work by slowing down how fast food travels through your gut, allowing stools to harden and solidify. The most popular antimotility drug is loperamide. Others include kaolin-and-morphine and co-phenotrope.

- **Linaclotide (Constella).** NICE also now recommends the

drug linaclotide (licensed in Europe in 2012) for IBS-related constipation, but only if other laxatives have already been tried at optimal or maximum doses and then only if the patient has had constipation for at least 12 months. Linaclotide works directly in the gut by binding to receptors in the gut wall, reducing pain and increasing the amount of fluid in the bowel so stools are loosened and move faster through the body. Other treatments for constipation include magnesium salts, and prucalopride, which is recommended by NICE for treating chronic constipation in women who have tried other laxatives and these haven't been effective.

13. Learn bio feedback

This is an outpatient service offered by some hospitals which trains patients to improve their own health by using signals from their own bodies. IBS patients are shown how to sit on the toilet, relaxing their muscles and slouching forwards with forearms on the lap. Later they lie down on a bed and a small balloon is inserted in to the back passage and inflated so the patient feels like they need to open their bowels. They are then told to push the balloon and the nurse can observe how they use their muscles and teach a more effective method.

14. Try psychological therapies

You may be resistant to the idea of using psychological therapies – perhaps you feel that your doctor is in some ways dismissing your symptoms as psychological or 'all in your mind', for instance, and can't see how seeing a psychological therapist can help you with very real physical gut problems. But as we've mentioned earlier in the book, the gut has a close connection with the brain (the so-called gut-brain axis) and also has its own enteric nervous system, plus research has shown that IBS sufferers are also more likely to suffer from anxiety and depression. NICE recommends psychological interventions (cognitive behavioural therapy [CBT], hypnotherapy and/or psychological therapy) should be considered for people with IBS who do not respond to pharmacological treatments after 12 months and who develop a continuing symptom profile (described as refractory IBS).

- **Cognitive behavioural therapy (CBT).** CBT is a talking therapy which teaches you how to interpret your symptoms differently and change the way you feel about them, in the hope of breaking the vicious circle of negative emotions provoking symptoms and vice versa. Increasingly it is prescribed as a computerised online treatment.[29]

- **Mindfulness.** Mindfulness is currently very fashionable – it's an integrative mind/body-based therapy that enables you to change the way you feel and think about experiences, especially stressful ones. According to Oxford University's Mindfulness Centre, mindfulness is about learning to enjoy living in the moment and paying attention to thoughts, feelings and body sensations to become directly aware of them. A 2013 study[30] in Calgary, Canada, found a course of mindfulness was beneficial to patients with IBS when followed up six months after their treatment had ended, compared with those who received standard treatment.

- **Counselling and psychotherapy** These psychological techniques help you deal with unresolved difficult life experiences or current situations that are making you ill, and are available via GP referral or privately. These issues may date back to childhood or be more recent.

15. Consider amitriptyline or other low-dose tricyclic anti-depressants

Studies have shown that antidepressants in low doses can improve IBS symptoms. NICE recommends tricyclic antidepressants

(TCAs), such as amitriptyline, as a second-line treatment for people with IBS if laxatives, loperamide or antispasmodics have not helped. They are only recommended for their pain-killing effects in IBS. NICE says the dose should be started at 5 to 10 mg a day and amitriptyline should be taken at night as it can be sedating. It should be regularly reviewed and the dosage increased if needed, but should not exceed 30 mg. NICE says selective serotonin reuptake inhibitors (SSRIs), such as Prozac, should only be prescribed if TCAs are not effective. If prescribed SSRIs, patients should be followed up after four weeks and then every six months.[31]

16. Try probiotics

There are 10 times as many bacteria in our gut as there are cells in our body and they play an important part in the body's immune system. The human microbiota (the technical name given to all the organisms living in the gut) consists of trillions of organisms from about 1,000 species.

Probiotics are live microorganisms which, when administered in sufficient quantities, may confer a benefit on the host. The most convincing evidence to date that bacteria may play a part in IBS is the finding that some susceptible individuals develop IBS after a bout of gastroenteritis. Current thinking is that abnormal changes in the gut microbiota lead to an immune response which increases gut permeability and dysregulates the enteric nervous system.[32]

Babies are born with sterile intestines but these are almost instantly colonised by bacteria from their mother's vagina and gut. Breast milk also contains prebiotics, which can help so-called 'friendly' bacteria thrive and build up a baby's immune system in the first two years of life. Industrialisation has been shown to change the gut microbiota – the Western diet with its high content of wholegrain cereals and resistant starch has been said to have profoundly altered the gut microbiota.

Some studies have found certain probiotic strains of 'friendly' bacteria (often sold as live yoghurt strains) may help reduce IBS symptoms, particularly bloating and diarrhoea.[33] The theory is that probiotics may improve intestinal barrier function and enhance the immune response against pathogens. There are numerous studies which have shown probiotics may be beneficial in improving IBS symptoms.[34, 35, 36, 37, 38]

One review of 16 randomised controlled trials on the safety and tolerability of probiotics in IBS patients published in 2009 found the strain *B. infantis 35624* was the only probiotic to have significant benefit. (PMID 19277023).[39] A review of 19 studies on the use of probiotics and IBS published in 2013[40] found that between 18 and 80 per cent of IBS patients responded to probiotics compared to between 5 and 50 per cent for placebo. A review published in the *World Journal of Gastroenterology* in 2015[41] found probiotics may significantly reduce pain in IBS – though these effects were weaker at follow-up in week 10 than they were in week 8, suggesting that they may have reduced effectiveness with long-term use.

The difficulties arise in distinguishing exactly which strains of probiotics are effective and what strength of supplement is needed to confer a benefit. According to a Yale University workshop[42] there are two types of probiotics which have the highest ratings for effectiveness: *Bifodobacterium infantis* 35624 and VSL#3. A study of 122 patients by the University of Milan in 2011[43] concluded the *Bifidobacterium bifidum* MIMbb75 probiotic strain improved IBS symptoms and quality of life compared to a placebo and was a 'promising treatment for IBS'. Another 2014 study indicated that all nine lactobacillus strains were able to survive in the gastrointestinal tract and 'could be considered good candidates for treatments and prevention of infections'.[44] But the upshot is that more trials are needed to determine which strains of bacteria may be most effective, what dosage is needed and to clarify whether a single strain or combination of different strains is needed.

In England NICE recommends patients who choose to try probiotics be given a month's trial while monitoring the effects. The main types of bacteria used in probiotic supplements are *Lactobacillus* and *Bifidobacterium*. The main drawback seems to be that the quality of supplements can vary as they are classed as foods and not medicines and not subject to the same quality controls, but experts agree they won't do you any harm and may be beneficial in some cases. It appears that they may be more effective on a single symptom rather than on all of them.

Scientists have used faecal transplants, where faecal bacteria from a healthy individual are transferred to a recipient whose gut microbiota has been disrupted, to successfully treat patients with recurrent infections of the 'super bug' *Clostridium difficile*, which causes diarrhoea. In the future it has been suggested that prebiotics (non-digestible carbohydrates that act as food for prebiotics), probiotics and faecal transplants might all be used to treat inflammatory bowel disease, obesity and type 2 diabetes.[45]

17. Hypnotise your gut

Bowel-directed hypnotherapy is an approach based on muscular and mental relaxation. General hypnotic suggestions are used to focus on or distract you from symptoms. Patients are encouraged to use the warmth of their hand resting on their abdomen to calm down areas of spasm and relieve pain. The concept is that you visualise your gut as a river and can slow it down or speed it up depending on whether you have constipation or diarrhoea. In 1984, Professor Peter Whorwell and colleagues in Manchester carried out a study[46] which found 80 per cent of IBS patients treated with gut-directed hypnotherapy reported improvements in symptoms. More recent randomised controlled studies carried out in Sweden[47] in 2012 found that whilst gut-directed hypnotherapy was effective, it was less so if given in a local hospital setting as opposed to a specialised gastrointestinal unit. However, the authors of the Swedish study concluded the effects were as least as effective as some of the newer IBS drugs on the market and had the advantages of having none of their side effects. A 2014 review of all the best quality research trials[48] concluded 'the study provides clear evidence that hypnotherapy has beneficial short-term effects for refractory IBS (IBS that is resistant to treatment). But the authors called for more randomised controlled trials (RCTs) to evaluate the long-term efficacy of hypnotherapy and they pointed out that all the existing RCTs had been carried out on patients with refractory IBS and therefore cannot be generalised to all IBS patients. The general consensus at the moment seems to be that gut-directed hypnotherapy won't do you any harm and is at least as effective as some drug treatments and may be worth a try if your symptoms have not responded to other treatments, but more research is needed to see if this is an effective long-term treatment.

18. Have a healthy lifestyle
Research on Chinese students found low levels of exercise and suffering from anxiety may be risk factors for IBS. Smoking has also been shown to be associated with IBS symptoms. Tobacco is believed to irritate the lining of the intestine.[49]

19. Avoid 'diet' products
Many diet products contain the sweetener sorbitol, which is a FODMAP (see page 37)[50] and can make diarrhoea and bloating worse. You will find sorbitol in various foods advertised as sugar-free, including chewing gum, sweets and yoghurts, so avoid these products if possible.

20. Evaluate any complementary remedies
Many IBS sufferers swear by the effectiveness of complementary remedies, including homeopathic remedies, aloe vera and acupuncture, but the evidence supporting their use is poor. A Cochrane review[51] published in 2013 concluded that two

studies involving the homeopathic remedy asafoetida (a spice derived from the herb fennel) improved symptoms in 75 per cent of patients whose predominant symptom was constipation, compared with 45 per cent who reported improvement in the placebo group. The review authors said larger, more robust trials were needed to conclusively prove the effectiveness of these remedies. Cochrane reviews are systematic reviews of primary research in human health care and health policy and are internationally recognised as the highest standard in evidence-based health care. They investigate the effects of interventions for prevention, treatment, and rehabilitation (see http:// uk.cochrane.org/about-us for more information).

21. Try peppermint oil (enteric coated)
Peppermint oil (page 45) has an antispasmodic effect (relieves muscle spasms) and works by blocking calcium channels in the smooth muscle of the bowel, relieving abdominal pain. According to the American Academy of Family Physicians peppermint oil may provide short-term relief and appears to be work better than a placebo in trials. However, there are no studies investigating the effects of long-term use.

22. Give charcoal tablets a go
Activated charcoal (where charcoal is heated with gas in order to increase its surface area) has been used as a remedy for upset stomachs for hundreds of years and is still a popular remedy that you can buy over the counter from pharmacies. The basic premise is that the charcoal has a mesh-like structure which absorbs toxins and gases – so it may reduce bloating for instance. However, there isn't any high-grade scientific evidence saying charcoal tablets are effective in treating IBS and there are also some concerns that it shouldn't be taken if you are on prescription medication as it may affect how the drug is absorbed into your system.

23. Cut down on booze

As suggested above, alcohol can be a trigger for IBS in some people[54] This is because alcohol irritates the stomach lining and more acid is produced triggering stomach pain, diarrhoea and vomiting. Keep within the recommended safe drinking limits of no more than 14 units of alcohol a week and if you know even small amounts upset your stomach, avoid it completely.

24. Get tested for coeliac disease and investigated for non coeliac gluten sensitivity

You can read more about these conditions in chapter 4. Even if you test negative for coeliac disease it it still possible your symptoms could be caused by gluten sensitivity (see page 72).

Expert summary by Professor Julian Walters

We have devoted a whole chapter to IBS as we find that it is a condition which causes a lot of dissatisfaction with current methods of diagnosis and treatment. This is partly because IBS symptoms fluctuate – you think you may have found the solution, only for the problem to come back again!

A lot of people have had many tests with no satisfactory answer, which is dispiriting. IBS doesn't kill you, but the effects on your life can be major, preventing you from enjoying food, social activities and life in general. However, as I hope we have shown you, there has been a lot of recent progress in identifying what may be contributing to your symptoms.

Table 3.2 summarises some of the information we have discussed in this chapter on treating IBS.

Table 3.2 What to do for IBS

Symptom	Action
If you have pain and bloating, think whether you have high lactose, gluten and FODMAPs in your diet.	These are the major food components linked to these symptoms. Keep a food and symptom diary for a while. You can find a lot of information about each of these, and you do not need to exclude them completely. A dietitian should be able to help analyse and make sure your diet is adequate.
Be sure coeliac disease has been excluded (see Chapter 4)	There are very accurate blood tests now.
If diarrhoea is the main problem, then bile acids may be the answer. Or possibly microscopic colitis (see Chapter 5)	Ask about getting tested for bile acid malabsorption /diarrhoea and current treatments for this common condition. Were biopsies taken at colonoscopy?
If constipation is the main problem, are you having enough bulk and osmotic laxatives? (see Chapter 9)	Try more fruit, vegetables, fibre, and possibly magnesium salts. But be aware of bloating, gas and FODMAPs.
General IBS symptoms	Have you had previous surgery or other treatment such as for cancer? Did these problems start when you went on to a new medicine? Think whether any previous disease or treatment could be linked to the symptoms.

Make sure that if your symptoms continue to affect you, you have considered all the issues identified in Table 3.2. Your GP or local dietitian can help you work your way through these, and provide medical and dietary advice. Although most people would prefer to find a dietary change that works, there are medicines that have some benefit for pain and bloating. If your pain is helped by amitriptyline for instance, it is perfectly fine to continue with that for many years. Loperamide can help prevent bowel urgency if you have to fly or go to the theatre. Fibre supplements provide you with a known amount of fibre that can reduce your needs from your diet, and should be thought of as food rather than medicine.

Excess of foods that may help some people can be the problem in others. The awareness of FODMAPs explains why fibre helps some but not many people with IBS. Advice to eat plenty of fruit and vegetables can lead to too much gas, liquid stools and discomfort. And we are starting to know much more about how colonic fermentation of these poorly absorbed foods changes intestinal bacteria (at least while you stay on these foods), and how your bacteria affect many aspects of how the intestine works, including fluid absorption, muscle and nerve function, and even hormones and immunity.

Get advice from experts. There are so many sources online to think about, and it can be confusing to balance the hype from the known facts and novel advances. Pharmaceutical companies have tried to come up with new medical approaches to 'IBS', but as many different processes can contribute to these symptoms, one size will not fit all – even if IBS is split into diarrhoea- or constipation-predominant.

Keeping a symptoms diary, learning about food and psychological triggers, managing stress and practising relaxation techniques, using medication, plus seeing your doctor for tests and a diagnosis can all help you manage your symptoms. It's important not to give up and keep trying new approaches until you find something that works for you.

Chapter 4

Coeliac disease and non-coeliac gluten sensitivity (NCGS)

Symptom checker

- Bloating
- Smelly diarrhoea
- Stomach pains / cramping
- Tiredness / fatigue
- Constipation
- Concentration problems

Is it gluten that's causing your gut problems?

It is fashionable to blame bread, pasta and other starchy carbohydrates for everything from stomach pains and diarrhoea to bloating and wind. Carbs seem to be the new bogeyman of the 21st century, just as saturated fat was in the late 20th century.

Celebrities and sportsmen and women are queuing up to tell us about how avoiding wheat has made them slimmer/less bloated/have more energy. Tennis player Novak Djokovic made headlines in 2011 when he put his success down to ditching pasta, bread and processed foods containing gluten. Carole Middleton, mother of HRH the Duchess of Cambridge, was reported to have famously slimmed down after following the no-carb Dukan diet before her daughter married Prince William in 2012.

But unlike most urban myths there's actually a grain of truth in carbs causing gut problems – at least in some people. This is because many of them contain gluten (proteins found in wheat, barley and rye), ingredients used to make bread and pasta and processed food, and gluten has been shown to trigger gut symptoms in certain susceptible individuals. In 2014, no fewer than 22 per cent of Americans interviewed for one survey said they were currently following a gluten-free diet – and as gluten-free foods are substantially more expensive than those containing gluten these people presumably did have gut-related symptoms they rightly or wrongly associated with foods containing gluten.[1] Another review of studies found that gluten is blamed by 20 to 45 per cent of adults who self-report food hypersensitivity.[2]

The difficulty is that there's lots of confusion: people often refer to themselves as having a 'wheat allergy' or 'sensitivity', or say they must follow a gluten-free diet, although they may have never had a medical diagnosis to confirm it. There are obvious dangers to this – by cutting out whole food groups on a whim you could deprive yourself of important nutrients, including B vitamins and fibre, and suffer constipation, tiredness and anaemia as a result. So if you suspect foods containing gluten are causing your symptoms it's important you see your doctor before you do anything else. Also, as we've discussed in Chapter 1, there are lots of other non-gluten related causes of bloating, including constipation, IBS, eating foods with a high FODMAP content and even just simple lifestyle issues, such as swallowing too much air while eating or drinking too many fizzy drinks. At the other end of the spectrum, bloating can also be one of the symptoms of ovarian cancer.

This chapter is designed to help you identify what the root cause of your symptoms might be, but it's not intended as a substitute for a diagnosis – symptoms such as persistent bloating / diarrhoea and abdominal pain should be checked out by your doctor.

Coeliac disease

An estimated 1 per cent of the population do have a genuine problem with foods containing gluten because they have coeliac disease, where the body's immune system mistakes gluten, a protein found in wheat, barley and rye, as a pathogen and their bodies mount an antibody response to it, damaging the finger-like projections on the lining of the gut called villi. These villi increase the surface area of the gut and make it easier for the body to absorb nutrients – so if they are damaged and become smaller you will not be able absorb nutrients from food as well as people who do not have coeliac disease.

Coeliac disease was identified as long ago as 1887 by Samuel Gee and in the 1930s and '40s the author of an influential paper on wheat and coeliac disease, WH Dicke, demonstrated that a diet free of wheat was key to avoiding damage to the gut and stopping the symptoms. In 1960 the first blood test for a serological marker for coeliac disease was discovered.[3]

Coeliac disease makes absorption of nutrients difficult and can lead to long-term complications, including anaemia and tiredness, osteoporosis (a fragile bone condition), unexplained infertility and a slightly higher risk of developing certain cancers and lymphomas if left undiagnosed and untreated.

Is it genetic?

There are genetic variants that have been identified as being associated with coeliac disease. The main link is with certain HLA types, known as dq2 or dq8. HLA stands for human leukocyte antigen, a gene which helps your body distinguish between its own proteins and those made by foreign bodies or invaders such as viruses and bacteria. If you have either of two versions of these genes, it's possible your body may mistake gliadin (and the other proteins found in gluten) as an invader and mount an immune response to it. This will cause inflammation in the intestine and lead to the symptoms of coeliac disease. However, it's not quite as simple as that. Although almost all people with coeliac disease have one of these genes, so do around 30 per cent of the population, and only 3 per cent of these have coeliac disease.[4] Clearly there must be other factors which may trigger coeliac disease. Some other genes have certain variants which make being a coeliac slightly more common. If you have a first-degree relative with the disease, your risk of being coeliac is up to 10 per cent (75 per cent if your identical twin has it) and you're also at higher risk if you have diabetes, other autoimmune diseases or Down's syndrome.[5]

Coeliac disease is *not* just a wheat allergy or intolerance though (see page 34). It's a lifelong autoimmune disease where the body's immune system attacks gluten and so damages the lining of the gut. To be free of symptoms and damage to the lining of your gut you have to avoid gluten for the rest of your life. Contrary to popular myth, you don't 'grow out of it' as you get older and it doesn't only affect white Caucasians either, but all racial groups. Prevalence does vary though – one recent European study found 2 per cent of people in Finland were coeliac compared to 0.3 per cent in Germany, for example.[6] The highest prevalence in the world is in the west of Ireland.[7]

Experts describe it as an 'iceberg disease' because the majority of cases are undiagnosed and below the water line; in the UK, for instance, it's estimated that around 75 per cent of cases are undiagnosed – that's around 500,000 people. Globally it's estimated that only 10 to 15 per cent of cases are diagnosed. Delayed diagnosis is common and researchers have shown that it takes 13 years on average to get a diagnosis.[8]

What makes coeliac disease difficult to diagnose?

Just about everything about coeliac disease makes it difficult to diagnose unless the right tests are done. It can have mild to severe symptoms, or no symptoms at all, and those symptoms can vary hugely and can be confused with other common conditions, including IBS (see Chapter 3, page 26).

We have said earlier in the book that myths about coeliac disease persist; people still wrongly believe it's rare, only happens in childhood and just affects white Caucasians living in Europe and North America – none of which is true. Coeliac disease can develop in adults and is common in North Africa, the Middle East, India and Pakistan, and recent studies suggest it is not uncommon in China.

Doctors may also struggle with spotting the symptoms, believing that chronic diarrhoea is always the main symptom, for instance. Apart from the classic symptoms of diarrhoea, weight loss and tiredness, coeliac disease can also cause non-classic symptoms which can easily be confused with other conditions. These include chronic fatigue, abdominal pain and distension, unexplained iron-deficiency anaemia, chronic migraine, peripheral neuropathy (numbness and tingling in the arms and legs), folic acid deficiency, unexplained infertility, delayed onset of periods, possibly unexplained miscarriage, dermatitis herpetiformis (an autoimmune skin-blistering disease which causes severe itching and stinging),[9] and reduced bone density. Neurological symptoms can also be associated with coeliac disease, including headaches, migraine, depression, loss of coordination (ataxia), attention deficit hyperactivity disorder (ADHD) and recurrent seizures. These vaguer symptoms can sometimes result in misdiagnosis and delayed diagnosis.

To complicate matters even more, coeliac disease can be asymptomatic in some people with no symptoms that they notice at all. These patients are usually picked up via routine screening tests (after a family member has been diagnosed, for instance). Studies in families have shown that 50 per cent of newly diagnosed coeliac disease patients had no symptoms. However, this doesn't mean their gut hasn't been damaged – biopsies will reveal damage and many report a 'new normality' (feeling better) after starting on a gluten-free diet.[10]

Because coeliac disease is so difficult to spot, NICE has provided some guidelines on when to test – see Box 4.1.

Box 4.1 NICE guidelines on when to test for coeliac disease[11]

NICE suggests that serological testing for coeliac disease should be offered to:
- people with any of the following:
  - o persistent unexplained abdominal or gastrointestinal symptoms
  - o faltering growth
  - o prolonged fatigue
  - o unexpected weight loss
  - o severe or persistent mouth ulcers
  - o unexplained iron, vitamin B12 or folate deficiency
  - o type 1 diabetes, at diagnosis

---

o   autoimmune thyroid disease, at diagnosis

o   irritable bowel syndrome (in adults).

- first degree relatives of people with coeliac disease.

Consider serological (blood) testing for coeliac disease in people with any of the following:

- metabolic bone disorder (reduced bone mineral density or osteomalacia)
- unexplained neurological symptoms (particularly peripheral neuropathy or ataxia)
- unexplained subfertility or recurrent miscarriage
- persistently raised liver enzymes with unknown cause
- dental enamel defects
- Down's syndrome
- Turner's syndrome.

Is coeliac disease on the increase?

More cases of coeliac disease are being diagnosed than ever before, but until the 1980s it was regarded as rare and mainly affecting children. Since then it's become apparent that coeliac disease can develop at any age. It's also more common in women than men, with a ratio of 4 to 3. A recent study in the UK by the University of Nottingham based on 10,000 people between 1990 and 2011 found incidence of coeliac disease had increased four-fold over the period.[12] Some experts argue that this is partly due to greater awareness of symptoms and improvements in diagnostic tests, but others speculate that it is the result of eating more foods containing gluten (although humans have been eating large amounts of bread for many centuries). Whilst humans have existed for 2.5 million years, wheat, barley and rye grains were only introduced into our diet about 10,000 years ago, and there is one school of thought that says some of us are not well adapted for the amount of gluten we are now eating. Foods containing gluten are now dietary staples in many parts of the world and include bread, baked goods, pasta and noodles, as well as bulgur and couscous in the Middle East and North Africa. In Europe the mean consumption of gluten is 10 to 20 g per day, with some segments of the population eating more than 50 g a day.[13] Gluten is also added to many processed foods – and most of us are eating more of those too. Others have proposed that we are now eating more of the grains most likely to be 'toxic' to the immune system due to the selections of wheat varieties with higher gluten content over the past 10,000 years. They argue that we now eat less of the wheat varieties grown for thousands of years such as *Triticum monococcum* (the oldest and most primitive cultivated wheat) and more of those with a higher gluten content.

Another theory is the so-called 'hygiene hypothesis', which proposes the increasing prevalence of allergic and autoimmune diseases in developed countries is due to the reduction in the incidence of infectious diseases achieved by vaccinations, improvements in hygiene, antibiotics and our increasingly 'clean' indoor lifestyles. In short, our immune systems aren't challenged as much in our early years as they used to be.

Others argue that breastfeeding may be protective against coeliac disease, although the research on this isn't conclusive. Gastrointestinal infections, surgery and drugs, including interferon, have all been suggested as possible triggers for coeliac disease

Symptoms of coeliac disease

The symptoms of coeliac disease may include:

- bloating
- smelly diarrhoea (greasy, with a high fat content)
- stomach cramps
- constipation
- sudden weight loss (but not in all cases)
- flatulence
- vomiting (usually only in children).

Non-gut symptoms may include:
- mouth ulcers
- headaches
- tiredness and fatigue
- iron-deficiency anaemia
- slow growth in children/short stature
- vomiting (usually only in children)
- swelling of hands, feet, arms and legs caused by a build-up of fluid (oedema)
- tingling and numbness in the hands and feet
- hair loss
- depression
- osteoporosis
- adverse pregnancy outcomes
- skin changes: dermatitis herpetiformis is a skin manifestation of coeliac disease which causes a rash with red raised patches, often with blisters on the elbows, knees, shoulders, buttocks and face. Only a minority of coeliac patients have this (an estimated 3,300 people in the UK according to the charity Coeliac UK).

Diagnosing coeliac disease

If you suspect you have coeliac disease it's really important you see your doctor *before* you start cutting out foods with gluten and going on a gluten-free diet. This is because coeliac disease can only be confirmed via a blood test for antibodies to gluten and a gut biopsy to check for damage to the lining of the gut – and if you are already avoiding gluten this may treat the condition and affect your results, making it appear you are not coeliac.

The gold standard for diagnosing coeliac disease according to the World Gastroenterology Organisation guideline on coeliac disease published in 2012 is a blood test for a biomarker for the condition (see below) and an intestinal biopsy to confirm damage to the gut (the technical name for this is villus atrophy).[14] A blood test alone cannot be relied upon, as between 6 and 22 per cent of all cases of coeliac disease are seronegative (they don't show up in blood tests).

With children, however, the guidelines recommend that those with the symptoms of coeliac disease don't need a biopsy to confirm their diagnosis if blood tests have revealed a high level of antibodies and they also have the genes (HLA types) of coeliac disease.[15]

What does a blood test look for?

Blood tests for coeliac disease look for antibodies produced by the body to gluten.

NICE guidance recommends immunoglobulin A (IgA) and IgA tissue transglutaminase (tTG) as the first choices for testing for suspected coeliac disease. It recommends IgA endomysial antibodies (EMA) if IgA tTG is weakly positive and to consider using IgG EMA, IgG deamidated gliadin peptide (DGP) or IgG tTG if IgA is deficient.

Although home test blood kits are available for coeliac disease, and these can provide the first clue that you might be a coeliac, the only way you can be definitely diagnosed is by a health professional and a positive blood test result, and this will still need confirming with a follow-up gut biopsy.

If you test positive for these antibody biomarkers, your GP should refer you on to a gastroenterologist to discuss further investigations, including a gut biopsy which will be done via a simple upper endoscopy (see Glossary). Even if you test negative for these antibody markers, your GP may still decide to refer you on to a gastroenterologist if your symptoms are suggestive of coeliac disease.[16]

Biopsies

If your blood tests are positive (or even in some cases if they are negative but your symptoms persist and are suggestive of coeliac disease) you should be referred to a gastroenterologist for a gut biopsy (see Glossary, page 180).

It's essential that you continue to eat gluten whilst you are waiting for this biopsy to be done for the reasons explained above. NICE recommends that patients should be advised to eat some gluten in more than one meal a day for a minimum of six weeks before the biopsy.[17]

According to World Gastroenterology Organisation guidelines, at least four biopsy samples should be taken from specific areas of the gut for lab analysis (and the authors point out it's really important the laboratory processing the test results has the relevant expertise and experience needed to interpret the results).[18]

Your gastroenterologist will then classify your biopsy results according to a classification called the Marsh Guidelines. The charity Coeliac UK has simplified these (see Table 4.1).

Table 4.1 Marsh Guidelines used for biopsy analysis

Marsh 0	The lining of the intestine is normal and it's unlikely you have coeliac disease.
Marsh 1	Increased number of lymphocytes (small white blood cells that are involved in the body's immune system response to the disease) is seen, but there are normal villi.
Marsh 2	Increased number of lymphocytes, the depressions in the lining of the intestine are deeper than normal but normal villi length.
Marsh 3	The villi are becoming flattened.
Marsh 4	The villi are completely flattened.

Source: Coeliac UK (www.coeliac.org.uk) with permission.[19]

How effective is following a gluten-free diet?

The short answer is usually very effective. Approximately 70 per cent of patients report an improvement in their symptoms within two weeks after starting a gluten-free diet.[20] Sometimes it can take up to two years for your gut to heal completely though, so give it time. But strict adherence is needed – eating just tiny amounts of gluten can cause symptoms to flare up again.

After your diagnosis you should automatically be referred to a dietitian for advice on which foods to avoid and those which are safe for you to eat (see Table 4.2). It's not as draconian as it sounds, especially nowadays when so many gluten-free foods are available, including gluten-free bread, cakes and ready meals – but it does require some vigilance and double-checking ingredients on packaging. You'll usually feel so much better, though, that you won't mind.

Table 4.2 Your gluten-free checklist

Grains to avoid	Grains that are safe	Other safe foods
Barley Bran Bulgur Couscous Durum flour Malt, malt extract, malt syrup Oat, oat bran, oat syrup (oats are tolerated by most (95 per cent) of coeliacs but the risk is that of cross contamination from other grains).	Amaranth Arrowroot Buckwheat Bean flours Corn Garbanzo beans Millet Montina flour Nut flour Oats (uncontaminated with rye or wheat) Seeds	Milk, cream, buttermilk, plain yoghurt All fresh meats Eggs Legumes (lentils, chickpeas, peas, beans, nuts and seeds) Fruits (fresh, frozen and canned fruits and plain juices. Vegetables (fresh, frozen and canned with no added and plain juices.
Rye Semolina Spelt Wheat germ, wheat starch, wheat brain Any item with wheat in the name Kamut Farro Emmer Einkhorn	Potato flour/potatoes Quinoa Rice Sorghum flour Soy flour Tapioca Teff flour	Liquid vegetable oils Sweets including corn syrups, brown and white sugars, plain popcorn, nuts. Pure black pepper, vinegars (apple, cider, distilled white)

Source: World Gastroenterology Organisation, 2012.[21]

Because gluten is an ingredient in bread, pasta and baked goods such as cakes and biscuits it can be tricky to avoid at first – always check ingredients on packaging. Ordering in restaurants is easier now because restaurants are now legally obliged to list gluten-free options.

The charity Coeliac UK provides an up-to-date directory of gluten-free food and drinks to members. For more details go to https://www.coeliac.org.uk/gluten-free-diet-and-lifestyle/food-and-drink-directory/

Some gluten-free foods are also available on NHS prescription – ask your GP about eligibility.

After your diagnosis, your dietitian should give you advice about how to get enough fibre in your diet as a gluten-free diet is typically low in fibre. Eating enough vegetables, including potatoes and perhaps also wholegrain rice, is very important to replace the roughage you'd normally get from wheat, barley and rye. You may also need vitamin or other supplements for the first few months at least to address any deficiencies in iron or folic acid.

What if your symptoms persist on a gluten-free diet?

The vast majority of people who have coeliac disease do find their symptoms go away when they go gluten-free, but in some cases, symptoms persist. Experts say this is nearly always due to eating gluten accidentally in some form – usually due to cross-contamination from a restaurant kitchen or a food processing plant or from an unexpected source such as postage stamps, lipstick, lip balm, tea bags (the glue round the edge) or some medicines.

You must be vigilant in your home when preparing your food too – by keeping kitchen cooking utensils apart, using separate bread boards for breads containing gluten and non-gluten breads and individual pots of butter, jam etc. to avoid cross contamination if you have non-coeliacs in the household.

In a tiny minority of cases, though, symptoms do not improve even when a gluten-free diet is strictly followed. There are three possibilities here – either you have developed secondary lactose intolerance (which is usually temporary), been misdiagnosed (in which case you may be referred for another biopsy) or you may have 'refractory coeliac disease'.

Secondary lactose intolerance is common after a coeliac diagnosis because damaged villi in the gut can mean that production of an enzyme called lactase needed to digest lactose (a sugar found in milk and dairy) is disrupted. This is usually temporary and once the villi heal, lactase should be produced normally again so you will be able to digest lactose – but this can take months or years. Because lactose is not broken down it moves on through the gut causing bloating, pain and diarrhoea. If you have been following a gluten-free diet and your symptoms have not improved you may want to ask your doctor about cutting out cow's milk and dairy products to see if it makes a difference.

Only an estimated one in 140 people with coeliac disease have **refractory coeliac disease** where, for reasons not fully understood, following a gluten-free diet has no effect on symptoms – or it works initially and then later no longer has any effect. It is rare under the age of 30 and more common in the over 50s. Symptoms include persistent severe diarrhoea, abdominal pain and weight loss. If a diagnosis of refractory coeliac disease is made the treatment options may include steroids, immunosuppressant drugs and chemotherapy or a combination of these drugs. There are two types of refractory coeliac disease and one of them has a higher risk of gut cancers.

You may also be advised to have vaccinations to strengthen your immune system, including the 'flu jab and vaccinations against Hib/Men C and pneumococcal disease.

A vaccine to 'cure' coeliac disease

A vaccine for coeliac disease is already in development and in clinical trials although these still have a long way to go before we know whether this approach could be effective. NETVAX2 works by reprogramming the body's immune system so that it doesn't attack the gut in response to gluten in the diet. It's been specially developed for use as a desensitisation vaccine treatment for the gene HLA DQ2 associated coeliac disease. Other vaccines are also in development.

Could you have non-coeliac gluten sensitivity (NCGS)?

What if you test negative for coeliac disease in blood tests and biopsies but still have some of the classic symptoms? This is a mystery that has puzzled gastroenterologists for years. Why do they see so many patients who complain of bloating, diarrhoea and stomach pain after eating foods such as bread and pasta, but who test negative for coeliac disease? And more importantly, why do many appear to get better when they switch to a gluten-free diet?

In the past if you tested negative for coeliac disease and still had symptoms you were told you simply didn't have coeliac disease and to just get on with it, but some gastroenterologists began to notice that some of these patients *did* get better if they switched to a gluten-free diet. A significant number of gastroenterologists now believe that these patients do actually have a medical condition: it's called non-coeliac gluten sensitivity (NCGS). It was first described in 1986. It has similar symptoms to coeliac disease, but does not appear to involve the immune system (so no antibodies show up on blood tests) or damage the lining of the gut, so biopsies are clear.

Crucially though, the symptoms of NCGS appear to go away if patients avoid foods containing gluten. Some studies suggest gluten may be reintroduced after following a gluten-free diet (a period of six months was suggested), suggesting patients try cereals with a low gluten content to begin with e.g. oats and einkorn farro (*Triticum monococcum*).[22]

Not all doctors believe NCGS exists as a well-defined, separate condition – mainly because no one understands what causes it and there is no diagnostic test for it as yet, but also because it's possible that symptoms get better due to the placebo effect. Others say there is considerable overlap with IBS. But NCGS is now gaining wider acceptance, mainly due to a flurry of new research in the last three years – and doctors say this has been driven by patients. Gastroenterologists say they have seen pictures of their patients' bloated bellies photographed on mobile phones shortly after eating gluten, for instance, and patient forums on the internet are abuzz with NCGS too, with people comparing their symptoms and the solutions they have come up with.

In November 2012, Dr Kamran Rostami wrote an article in the *British Medical Journal*[23] describing a patient who had been troubled by abdominal pain, diarrhoea, bloating, joint pain, fatigue and many other symptoms. He tested negative for coeliac disease but his health improved dramatically after he switched to a gluten-free diet.

Dr Rostamai wrote: 'It's now becoming clear that, besides those with coeliac disease or wheat allergy, there are patients with gluten sensitivity in whom neither allergic nor autoimmune mechanisms can be identified. It has been estimated that, for every person with coeliac disease, there should be at least six or seven people with non-coeliac gluten sensitivity. Gluten sensitivity may therefore affect 6–10% of the general population. This means approximately 4–7 million people in the United Kingdom have this condition, and the vast majority are unaware of their sensitivity to gluten.'

After the article was published, Dr Rostami received scores of emails from doctors and patients wanting to know more about NCGS. Since then there has been a clutch of new articles published in international medical journals attempting to define NCGS, but due to the lack of a biological marker (no reliable test for NCGS has yet been identified) this is regarded as a limitation of clinical studies.

One paper[24] described NCGS as a combination of IBS-like symptoms (including abdominal pain, bloating, bowel habit abnormalities) and systemic manifestations, including 'foggy' mind, headaches, fatigue, joint and muscle pain, leg or arm numbness, dermatitis, depression and anaemia. The symptoms in NCGS may resemble those associated with coeliac disease but with a prevalence of other symptoms, such as behavioural changes, bone or joint pain, muscle cramps, leg numbness, weight loss and chronic fatigue.

Between 2004 and 2010, 5,896 patients were seen at the Center for Celiac Research, University of Maryland. The criteria for GS (NCGS) were fulfilled by 347 (1:17; 6 per cent) of the patients seen. Their symptoms included abdominal pain (68 per cent); eczema and/or rash (40 per cent); headache (35 per cent);

'foggy mind' (34 per cent); fatigue (33 per cent); diarrhoea (33 per cent); depression (22 per cent); anaemia (20 per cent); numbness in the legs, arms or fingers (20 per cent); and joint pain (11 per cent).[25]

Experts say the overall prevalence of NCGS is still unknown mainly because most patients diagnose themselves and start a gluten-free diet without medical advice or consultation. In a study amongst children who were non-coeliacs in New Zealand, 5 per cent were following a gluten-free diet. Another US study put the figure for NCGS at nearer 0.5 per cent.

Other studies have identified a possible overlap with IBS; in Northern Europe prevalence of IBS is between 16 and 25 per cent and in one large study, for instance, 30 per cent of patients with IBS symptoms also suffered from wheat sensitivity.[26] A 2015 double blind randomised controlled trial found 25.7 per cent of IBS patients given a powder containing gluten reported an improvement in symptoms compared with 83.8 per cent given a gluten-free powder. The authors concluded a large number of patients labelled as having IBS are sensitive to gluten.[26A]

Latest theories put forward include the concept that it isn't the gluten in wheat that causes the sensitivity in NCGS patients at all, but other components such as FODMAPs (see Chapter 3, page 37). FODMAPS are found in wheat, some vegetables and milk products. One double blind randomised controlled trial (the gold standard method in medical research) carried out by Biesiekierski et al. found that IBS-like symptoms were more frequent in the gluten treated group (68 per cent) rather than in the placebo group (40 per cent).[27] A second study[28] found patients who self-reported with IBS/NCGS, and who were randomly assigned a low FODMAPs diet, reported their symptoms significantly improved and then worsened when put on a gluten/whey challenge.

Experts say the results raise the possibility that the positive effects of a gluten-free diet in patients with IBS is 'an unexpected consequence' of reducing FODMAPs, given wheat is a possible source'. However, other academics say it should be stressed that FODMAPs cannot be entirely and exclusively responsible for the symptoms experienced by NCGS subjects, since their symptoms disappear while on a gluten-free diet despite continuing to eat FODMAPs from other sources, like legumes (a much richer source of FODMAPs than wheat).

In an article published in April 2015 in the *United European Journal of Gastroenterology*, Jessica Biesiekierski from the Translational Research Centre for GI Disorders in Belgium, the author of the two studies cited above, concluded, 'There is some evidence that NCGS may exist, but probably only in a small number of people.'[29] She said: 'Much of the confusion and controversy has arisen in part from a failure to distinguish clearly between the gluten and fructan components of wheat.'

She continued: 'Indeed, patients who believe they have NCGS are likely to benefit from lowering their dietary intake of FODMAPs. Providing the careful design of clinical trials, the next several years will provide a stronger quality of evidence and exciting key pieces to understand this NCGS puzzle.'

What should you do if you think you have NCGS?

The current advice is to carry on eating foods containing gluten at least until you can get tested for coeliac disease. If you have already had the blood tests and biopsy for coeliac disease and both are negative, ask your gastroenterologist about a trial of either a gluten-free-diet or a low FODMAPs diet. New guidelines on diagnosing NCGS were published in 2015 (the Salerno Experts' Criteria); ask your doctor about following a double-blind placebo-controlled gluten challenge.[30]

Case study

Sue C, a woman in her 50s from London, was recently diagnosed with NCGS, after suffering from bloating, fatigue and diarrhoea since the age of eight. Sue had been told she had a 'grumbling appendix' as a child when she suffered tummy cramps. Later she was told it was irritable bowel syndrome that was to blame and told to eat a high-fibre diet which made her symptoms worse. In her 30s her GP just dismissed her symptoms as signs of stress.

But after seeing a gastroenterologist two years ago and testing negative for coeliac disease, Sue was eventually diagnosed with NCGS and switched to a gluten-free diet. Now her symptoms have disappeared. She's got her energy back, has lost two stone and has no more stomach pain or diarrhoea. She just wishes she'd been diagnosed years ago.

The worrying thing is that there could potentially be millions of people just like Sue in the UK.

Wheat allergies and intolerances

A wheat allergy is where the immune system reacts to proteins found in wheat and this usually happens within a few seconds/minutes of eating. It's uncommon and involves the body making a type of antibody (IgE) to fight off a suspected 'invader' – in this case some of the proteins found in wheat. When the food is next eaten, or sometimes if it just comes into contact with the skin, it triggers a full-blown response from the immune system and the release of histamine, a chemical which causes inflammation in the body leading to symptoms such as asthma, wheezing, a runny nose, itchy rash, as well as diarrhoea, stomach pains and worsening of eczema. This usually happens a few seconds or minutes after exposure to the protein. It is similar to a shellfish or peanut allergy. In the most serious cases, anaphylaxis, a severe life-threatening form of allergic response, can result. It can be treated with an injection of adrenaline to dampen down the inflammatory response and steroids. Doctors diagnose it with a blood test for antibodies or a pinprick skin test.

However, in children it's possible to have a delayed allergic response to wheat, with symptoms developing within 24/48 hours and then it can be more difficult to work out what has caused the reaction. After repeated exposure, the child may be failing to put on weight, have worsening eczema and suffer diarrhoea.

Most people who say they have a wheat allergy don't have an allergy at all but an intolerance – which doesn't involve the immune system. The symptoms come on more slowly than the classic wheat allergy symptoms within several hours and include bloating, cramps, diarrhoea and sickness and there's no diagnostic test as no antibodies are produced. If these symptoms are troubling you, ask your GP for a referral to a dietitian for advice – they may advise you to keep a food diary of your symptoms to identify the foods that are troubling you and then try eliminating them, and rechallenging yourself with the food later. More recently, the effects of a low FODMAPs diet have been found to be useful in these circumstances.[31]

Chapter 5

Watery diarrhoea

Watery diarrhoea all the time? Smelly wind and painful cramps? You could have bile acid diarrhoea (BAD), small intestinal bacterial overgrowth (SIBO) or microscopic colitis.

Symptom checker

- Up to 10 bowel movements a day
- Watery, pale or foul-smelling stools
- Painful abdominal cramps
- Flatulence
- Urgency
- Incontinence (accidents) in some cases

Bile acid diarrhoea

Bile acid diarrhoea (BAD) isn't that well known, but some experts estimate as many as a third of the patients currently diagnosed with irritable bowel syndrome (IBS) with diarrhoea as the predominant symptom (IBS-D) could have it – that's at least one million people in the UK alone (based on nine million people having IBS in the UK).[1] You may never have heard of BAD – but that certainly doesn't mean it's rare. This is backed up by systematic review of scientific studies.[3]

It seems incredible that so many people may have this condition but no one has heard of it, even though dozens of scientific papers have been written on it dating back 35 years; experts say the difficulties lie in the lack of a widely available diagnostic test – but also just a general lack of awareness amongst both doctors and the general public.

BAD is also called bile acid malabsorption (BAM) or bile salt malabsorption (BSM). It is a type of diarrhoea caused by bile salts produced by the liver not being produced or recycled properly. Normally 95 per cent of bile salts are absorbed at the end of the small intestine and less than 0.5 g of bile acids enter the colon daily. In BAD the excess bile passes into the colon, stimulating electrolyte (salts) and water secretion, which results in chronic watery diarrhoea. It is often overlooked and under-diagnosed and patients can struggle on with the symptoms for year after year without ever getting a diagnosis or treatment.

Symptoms

BAD is every bit as nasty as it sounds; the symptoms may include up to 10 watery bowel movements a day, smelly wind, severe cramp-like pains in your abdomen, bloating, and an urgent need to get to a loo, and sometimes 'accidents' (faecal incontinence) when the sufferer doesn't make it in time. It can be very debilitating and leave some people effectively housebound as they dare not go too far from a toilet. When it's described in these terms it's surprising that many patients put up with these symptoms for many years and most never get the correct diagnosis.

It's common to meet patients who have had symptoms of diarrhoea for many years without an accurate diagnosis and specific treatment. Clinicians often don't recognise BAD as a cause of this disorder and might not perform investigations. Often doctors will just dismiss it as IBS. Patients' stories written up in medical journals tell of social embarrassment, loss of employment opportunities and repeated unnecessary investigations.

Symptoms that could be IBS are one of the most common reasons for referral to a gastrointestinal clinic and can account for up to one in 20 of the patients seen.[4] IBS is estimated to affect nine million adults in the UK; of those three million are estimated to have diarrhoea as the predominant symptom. However, the cause of the diarrhoea is often difficult to diagnose and patients may undergo several investigations, including those for inflammatory bowel disease, colonic cancer, coeliac disease and chronic infections, without a definitive cause being identified or effective treatment. It's common to meet patients who have had symptoms of diarrhoea for many years without an accurate diagnosis and specific treatment.

Why does it matter? Well, unlike IBS, there *is* a diagnostic test for BAD and effective drug treatments, so getting the correct diagnosis could save you many years of distressing symptoms. Professor Julian Walters, Professor of Gastroenterology at Imperial College, London, and one of the authors of this book, believes BAD is much more common than was previously thought and is frequently being wrongly diagnosed as IBS. He is passionate about getting it on the radar of more doctors and patients. Sometimes knowledgeable doctors do think about BAM, but only as the condition that some patients get after bowel surgery for Crohn's disease. A research study[5] which questioned 706 British gastroenterologists about bile acid malabsorption/diarrhoea found low awareness of the condition. Sixty per cent of the gastroenterologists who replied said that of 500 new patients referred to them, 34 per cent had diarrhoea and 1 per cent of them had been diagnosed with BAM. In those with chronic diarrhoea, only 6 per cent had been investigated for BAM as a first-line investigation and 61 per cent of gastroenterologists said they would consider the diagnosis only in selected patients.

Professor Walters says repeated studies suggest that as many as a third of all patients in the NHS who are currently treated for IBS-D (IBS where diarrhoea is the predominant symptom) actually have bile acid diarrhoea – and so BAD potentially affects huge numbers of people – more than diseases such as Crohn's and ulcerative colitis, which are much better known about. He says: 'Most patients and many doctors are unaware that bile acid diarrhoea even exists and that there is a diagnostic test and effective drug treatment available.'

One study of 62 patients with chronic watery diarrhoea and no obvious causes on initial investigation, found 45 per cent of the patients had bile acid diarrhoea, 16 per cent had coeliac disease, 16 per cent had gluten sensitivity and 20 per cent had no specific diagnosis.[6] Another review published in 2015 found that more than a quarter of patients with watery diarrhoea of unknown cause had BAD.[7]

What are bile acids and why do they cause a problem?

Bile acids are essential for digestion and absorption of fats and fat-soluble vitamins in the small intestine. The liver produces and passes large amounts of bile acids into the intestine every day, but only relatively small quantities are lost from the body. This is because approximately 95 per cent of the bile acids are recycled back to the liver from the ileum (the end part of the small intestine). But in bile acid diarrhoea, more bile acid is lost and the excess bile in the colon stimulates electrolyte (salts) and water secretion, which results in (chronic) watery diarrhoea.

Different types of bile acid diarrhoea

There are broadly three types of BAD. These include:

- **Type 1 BAD.** This happens as a result of either ileal resection (see Glossary) or ileal inflammation, such as that caused by Crohn's disease, a type of inflammatory bowel disease where any part of the gastrointestinal tract becomes ulcerated and bleeds (see Chapter 6).

- **Type 2 BAD/idiopathic/primary bile acid malabsorption.** This occurs when the BAD is not related to any other gut disorder. Recent research has found the trigger for type 2 BAD is actually a hormone disorder – deficiency of a hormone called fibroblast growth factor 19 (FGF19), which normally switches off bile production when bile is reabsorbed. In healthy people, when bile acid is absorbed by the intestine, the body makes more FGF19 to stop new bile from being produced, but in people with BAD, less FGF19 is produced so the hormone switch fails to turn off. The result is that more bile is produced than the intestine can absorb and the resulting watery secretions cause diarrhoea.

- **Type 3 BAD.** This can occur as a secondary complication to other gastrointestinal complaints, including small intestinal bacterial overgrowth (SIBO) (see page 92), coeliac disease, cholecystectomy (see Glossary, page 180), post radiation treatment for cancer and chronic pancreatitis (see Chapter 6, page 133).

Diagnosing bile acid diarrhoea

Lots of research has gone into trying to find a reliable diagnostic test for BAD. The SeHCAT test, which uses a selenium-labelled synthetic bile salt (see Glossary), was developed by scientists in

Edinburgh in the late 1980s and is now used at many specialist centres in the UK and Europe, but is not available in the US.

The technology is used, in conjunction with a full-body scan, to test the function of the bowel by measuring how well the compound is retained or lost from the body. In a person with normal bile acid function, more than 15 per cent of SeHCAT is detected in the body after seven days, having been reabsorbed over and over again, but in people with bile acid diarrhoea the percentage can be as low as 1 to 5 per cent.

Unfortunately, although the SeHCAT test is available, the UK's National Institute for Health and Care Excellence (NICE) has ruled that there is insufficient evidence 'at present' to determine whether it is a useful and cost-effective diagnostic test for people with idiopathic (primary/type 2) bile acid malabsorption. The NICE guidance therefore recommends that SeHCAT is used only in research settings in order that further evidence about its potential benefits for people with these conditions can be generated.

However, Professor Walters says that many clinical gastroenterologists who have become familiar with BAD and the use of SeHCAT were surprised how cautious this report was, given the weight of high quality research in this area, and he is concerned that many patients can go for years before the correct diagnosis is made. He says the SeHCAT test costs are less than those for having another colonoscopy or CT scan. About two-thirds of patients who test positive by SeHCAT will respond to the current drugs, but it can take time and persistence to adjust the dosage to generate an improvement in the symptoms. Some patients are very responsive but, although the diarrhoea is helped, pain from constipation can become a new problem. He states that both he and the patients are happier to have a definite diagnosis before beginning what can be long-term treatment.

He says demand for the test from clinicians in the UK has been remarkable and he is hoping the NICE guidelines might be updated soon. SeHCAT is not approved for use in the US and is not widely available in Europe either so the likelihood of it becoming a global test is small.

Blood and urine tests

Alternative tests that are being developed include a blood test for C4, a marker for increased bile acid synthesis, and another for the hormone FGF19. Researchers hope these will produce an easy, cheap way of diagnosing BAD and that targeting FGF19 production could result in new treatments being discovered. A urine test for volatile organic compounds which may also indicate the presence of abnormal bile acid levels is also being investigated.

Some gastroenterologists will offer a therapeutic trial of bile acid sequestrant medication (see page 85) without doing a diagnostic test to see if it is beneficial, although it's obviously preferable to get a diagnosis first.

Treatments for bile acid diarrhoea

Treatments for BAD were originally developed to treat high cholesterol and are called bile acid sequestrants. These drugs are positively charged with an indigestible resin that binds the bile acid in the intestine to form an insoluble complex that is then excreted in a stool.

There are three different types:
- Colestyramine (Questran): available as a powdered paste
- Colestipol: available as a powder in a sachet
- Colesevelam: available as tablets and said to be more palatable.

The effectiveness of the treatment is around 96 per cent for patients with the lowest SeHCAT scores (less than 5 per cent, and more serious BAD symptoms) and 70 per cent for those with milder forms of BAD with bile acid scores of less than 15 per cent. Unfortunately, the powdered medicines can have an unpleasant taste and patients have to make an effort to find a way to make them more palatable by mixing with certain foods and liquids (see Box 5.1).

All these treatments can have side effects and many patients don't tolerate them, with between 40 and 70 per cent discontinuing their treatment, reporting flatulence, bloating, nausea and abdominal discomfort. This can be due to the drug being *too* effective and producing these symptoms, including constipation.

Gastroenterologists advise starting on a low dose and gradually increasing it to minimise side effects – the majority of patients do tolerate the drugs when they are started on them in this way.

Box 5.1 Tips to make bile acid sequestrants more palatable

- Add powder to a half cup of water, fruit drink or juice and mix thoroughly
- Try mixing it with pudding or custard
- Add powder to a half cup of apple sauce, crushed pineapple or strained fruit baby food
- Add powder to half a cup of milk, refrigerate the mixture and stir well before drinking.

Source: Parrish, 2012[8]

What should you do if you suspect you have bile acid diarrhoea?

If you've read this chapter, and recognise the symptoms of BAD and feel they reflect your own symptoms which have persisted long term, see your doctor, ask whether you could have it and request a referral to a gastroenterologist. Be prepared to get over your embarrassment and talk about your stools and frequency of your diarrhoea bouts – if you're not honest about how bad your symptoms are, the chances are your doctor will take them less seriously. It may help if you keep a diary of your symptoms that you can take along to the consultation.

Case study 'It took more than 40 years to diagnose my bile acid diarrhoea'

One woman in her 60s, (let's call her Anne*) suffered from persistent diarrhoea all her adult life and was finally diagnosed in 2013 after reading about BAD and the SeHCAT test on the internet. Her problems started at the age of 21 while she was studying at university. Her story is similar to many patients. She described it as follows:

'The diarrhoea would be particularly bad after breakfast and I'd need to go to the toilet lots of times in the morning. There was no blood and it wasn't painful, but it made me feel exhausted. Commuting to work was difficult and I'd have to stop several times on my journey. I found meetings at work a problem as I would have to keep popping out to the loo. These symptoms had a big impact on my life and stopped me working at the jobs I wanted.

* Name has been changed to protect anonymity.

'When I went to my GP, several times they made referrals to specialists. The same investigations were repeated and I had several colonoscopies and gastroscopies, but these tests always showed nothing was wrong. I was told this must just be IBS, and that I should reduce the amount of stress in my life. But my life was not that stressful, and when I retired from work and could finally relax there was no change to the diarrhoea. I was still getting unpredictable urges to dash to the toilet, no matter what I ate or how I relaxed. I had to arrange my life around toilet stops – it meant I could never enjoy going out to eat as I knew it might cause repeated bouts of diarrhoea.

'After a particularly difficult time, I went on the internet and Googled "longstanding diarrhoea" to see what came up. I came across an article which talked about a scientific paper published by Professor Julian Walters, on a condition called bile acid diarrhoea (BAD) and how it is often misdiagnosed as irritable bowel syndrome (IBS). When I read his description of the condition, it immediately made sense – it was as if he was describing my symptoms in detail. I couldn't believe no doctor had ever mentioned this condition to me before. I emailed Professor Walters in London in desperation.

'I described my symptoms to him and he said it seemed likely that I could have BAD. I saw him in his out-patient clinic and he arranged a SeHCAT test. I had to make two trips to the hospital for this and I took a pill with the special test substance. I had a simple scan after a couple of hours and then came back a week later to have it repeated. This was no problem at all – except for having to travel to the hospital and worrying about whether I might have to find a toilet in a hurry.

'When I saw him to find out about the results, he said they were positive. After 40 years of unending problems with diarrhoea, I finally had a diagnosis. It was such a huge relief to know my problem was not "just IBS" and that there was something new to try. I started taking a powder called colestyramine and within a week found an improvement. My stools were much more solid and I didn't get the urgent need to go anymore. I do need to keep taking this, because if I forget it for a day or two, then my diarrhoea comes back.

'I want to help people find out about this disease as I now know there are many people suffering like I was. I want them to know that a test is available and that current treatments help a lot. Some people I have met have told me that they dislike taking bile acid sequestrants (colestyramine is one of these) but I think this is worth it as, in my case, they help a lot. Perhaps better treatments can be found and I am trying to help with the research studies that are now starting. However, just knowing the cause of my symptoms has helped greatly. I hope more people like me get the proper diagnosis.'

Small intestinal bacterial overgrowth (SIBO)

Small intestinal bacterial overgrowth is the medical term to describe the situation when there are too many bacteria present in the small intestine. The small intestine usually has only low numbers of bacteria (unlike the large intestine, where their concentration is at least a million times higher). In the large intestine, bacteria can be useful to the body, digesting unabsorbed foods like fibre and helping obtain further nutrients. However, if there are too many bacteria in the small intestine they can also produce symptoms (in a similar way to FODMAPs, see Chapter 3, page 35).

There are normally low numbers of bacteria in the small intestine, which helps prevent bacterial breakdown of the enzymes and bile salts needed for normal digestion. The body is usually very good at preventing a build-up of small intestinal bacteria. Acid in the stomach will kill any swallowed bacteria and normal peristalsis (the contractions of the gut to push food along it) will sweep any bacteria from the small intestine down towards the large intestine.

When the number of bacteria gets too high in the small intestine this then produces the condition which is often called SIBO (or sometimes small bowel bacterial overgrowth – SBBO.) Gastroenterologists have known about this condition for several decades, although it can be hard to diagnose. It is probably the next most common cause of malabsorption after coeliac disease. It can cause fatty stools, other types of diarrhoea, weight loss, bloating and often anaemia or other measurable effects of impaired absorption of foods.

Diagnosis can be made by collecting small intestinal juices (usually through an upper endoscopy) and culturing the bacteria. But it can be hard to get clear counts. Often when the condition is suspected, a trial of treatment with standard antibiotics improves the bowel symptoms, making the diagnosis likely. An alternative indirect test is a glucose hydrogen breath test (see Glossary, page 183).

Usually there is a clue that SIBO is a possible diagnosis as people have already had some sort of bowel problem. It is commoner in people with Crohn's disease (see Chapter 6, page 104) especially after surgery, or when people have had other abdominal surgery which may have affected the way peristalsis keeps the small intestine clear, perhaps by forming adhesions. Sometimes there is another disease which has already been diagnosed affecting nerve or muscle function or causing scarring. It can occur in cancer survivors who have had radiation or other treatment which may have caused scarring and changed intestinal motility. Reduced stomach acid may also be a factor, and many people are taking medicines such as proton pump inhibitors (PPIs) to try and achieve that. Diverticula (little pouches, see Chapter 9, page 175) in the small intestine can be a cause, but they are much rarer here than in the large intestine, where we nearly all will get some. These conditions all can prevent the normal processes working to keep the small intestinal bacterial counts low and SIBO is accepted by experts as a cause of symptoms in these conditions. But is it a more widespread issue?

SIBO has been in the news recently as a possible cause of IBS symptoms. Dr Mark Pimentel from Los Angeles has published several scientific papers looking at this possibility, and he has written a book on this theory and promoted antibiotic treatments.[9-11]

He used a different hydrogen breath test initially (with lactulose, a non-absorbed sugar often given as a laxative). It has been difficult to get full acceptance of this theory as early appearance of hydrogen after lactulose could be due to rapid transit as well as a possible SIBO. Antibiotics which are active in the gut, but are not absorbed, help people with SIBO, and have helped many IBS sufferers – at least for a short time. One of these is Rifaximin, which is not currently licensed in the UK for this. Usually symptoms returned a few weeks after the course of antibiotics so this approach is unlikely to be a permanent cure.

Whether non-absorbed antibiotics will become an accepted approach to treating IBS and chronic diarrhoea is far from certain, but this is definitely an area to watch.

Microscopic colitis

Microscopic colitis is another condition that you may not have heard about before and can be a cause of the chronic diarrhoea symptoms (urgency, incontinence, abdominal bloating or pain) described at the beginning of this chapter. Unlike SIBO, there is nothing controversial about this – it is just that it is relatively new and many people haven't heard about it.[12]

Microscopic colitis was first described in the 1980s in people with severe watery diarrhoea.[13] It is not ulcerative colitis or Crohn's colitis, both well-known inflammatory bowel diseases (IBD), conditions which we will describe in more detail in Chapter 6. Unlike IBD, there are no ulcers in the bowel, no bleeding or anaemia, and the mucosa (the inside lining of the colon) looks normal when a colonoscopy is done. It is only when biopsies are taken during colonoscopy, and slides made from them are looked at under the microscope, that the abnormalities are seen. There are two types – lymphocytic colitis, where there is an increased number of the lymphocyte white blood cell, and collagenous colitis. In collagenous colitis, there is a thick abnormal band of the protein collagen, which is usually found in skin and tendons, just below the otherwise normal colon cells. These changes are often found together. They presumably slow down water absorption from the stool and/or lead to more secretion, and so give the characteristic frequent, watery stools.

Microscopic colitis is reasonably common, affecting about one in 1000 people at any time point. This means it is not much rarer than ulcerative colitis. It is about three times commoner in women and peaks around the age of 60. It may be more frequent with some other auto-immune disorders like thyroid disease, coeliac or diabetes, and in people taking antacid medicines, such as proton pump inhibitors. There is a link with bile acid diarrhoea which is commoner in people with microscopic colitis, particularly if it is the collagenous colitis variant.

If you have persistent diarrhoea, this chapter should have persuaded you to get further investigations and advice. GPs are pretty good these days in referring people who have a change in bowel habit for investigations, which often include a colonoscopy. There is a catch here though: maybe you had a colonoscopy and were told: 'You are all right. Nothing to worry about. We didn't see anything nasty like a cancer, and you didn't have any polyps or colitis.'

You need to ask: 'Did you take any biopsies? Did they show any microscopic colitis?'

Unless the colonoscopist takes biopsies which are looked at under the microscope, you will not be certain whether microscopic colitis has been ruled out or not. Biopsies taken at full colonoscopy are slightly better than if they have been taken at sigmoidoscopy, but most cases should still be diagnosed. It is unfortunate, but sometimes the test needs to be repeated just to get some biopsies. About one in 10 colonoscopies done for watery diarrhoea, and which appears to be normal, is said to show microscopic colitis.

Microscopic colitis is usually now treated with a medicine called budesonide, in a controlled release form. Budesonide is a type of steroid that is safer than prednisolone as it is broken down in the liver as soon as it has been absorbed into the bloodstream. The controlled release means that it is delivered to the end of the intestine without being absorbed before then and so is able to act where it is needed in the colon. It is a bit like putting a steroid cream on your skin to just work there for a rash.

Usually people with microscopic colitis are treated for three months or so and their diarrhoea and other symptoms rapidly get better. After this course, many people do not have another episode for many years. Sometimes the diarrhoea returns quite quickly, but another few months of budesonide will work for this next time. It is worthwhile considering if any other medicines might be linked to the onset of the symptoms and changing these if possible. Some people need to stay on a dose of Budesonide for some years to control their symptoms. Some other medicines are sometimes used, but budesonide has been a big advance.[14]

Fortunately microscopic colitis can now be settled with this treatment fairly easily and it does not then seem to be a problem. There are unfortunately people who think they have had 'all the tests' but have not had colonic biopsies done to be sure that they do not have this condition.

Just like BAD, where people suffer with their symptoms for years before getting the correct test, people with microscopic colitis can suffer needlessly because they have not had biopsies. Be sure this is not you if you have persistent watery diarrhoea, urgency or are sometimes incontinent of runny diarrhoea.

Chapter 6

Inflammatory bowel disease

What is causing the growing number of cases of these painful and debilitating bowel diseases and how are they treated?

Symptom checker

- Diarrhoea (often with mucus, blood or pus)
- Colicky abdominal pain
- Tiredness and fatigue
- Feeling unwell
- Rectal bleeding
- Feeling of incomplete emptying of your bowels
- Mouth ulcers
- Loss of appetite
- Weight loss

Sometimes the following symptoms can occur too:
- Swollen joints
- Skin rashes/eyes problems/joint inflammation
- Abscesses and fistulas

What is inflammatory bowel disease?

Inflammatory bowel disease (IBD) is an umbrella term for diseases which cause either whole or part of the digestive tract to become sore and inflamed. It commonly starts in younger people aged 10 to 40, although younger and older people may be affected too. The two most common types of IBD are **Crohn's disease** (CD) and **ulcerative colitis** (UC); the symptoms for both can be similar but with some distinguishing characteristics (see below). In the 19th and 20th centuries prevalence of IBD increased with industrialisation and the highest rates in the world are still in developed countries such as the UK, Canada, the USA and Western Europe – although cases are now increasing in China and India (see below).

Crohn's disease may affect the whole digestive tract from your mouth to your anus; ulcerative colitis affects only the colon and rectum. Crohn's disease can be more serious as it not only affects the lining of the gut but can also extend deeper into the wall of the bowel and this sometimes results in severe complications. Both can be extremely painful and debilitating, leading to weight loss and fatigue, and have a great impact on your quality of life, affecting your ability to digest food and absorb nutrients from it, as well as the frequent trips to the toilet. They tend to flare up and then go into remission.

The IBD 'epidemic'

IBD cases have increased dramatically in the UK, Europe and the US to around twice the prevalence of 30 or so years ago and cases are also beginning to increase in other parts of the world, including China and India.[1] Once regarded as rare, this is no longer the case with IBD and some doctors have even referred to it as reaching 'near epidemic proportions'.[2] What's more, doctors still have no definitive answers as to why it is happening – although changes in diet, gut bacteria (microbiome), increasing industrialisation, smoking and improved hygiene in childhood offer some potential explanations. It's a particularly worrying trend because there appear to be more cases starting earlier in childhood (and IBD can be more severe in the childhood years), and it also means that people are more at risk of complications the longer they live with it.

Latest figures suggest there are now around 300,000 people with IBD diseases in the UK – and around 0.5 per cent of the population in the developed world.[3] This 2012 review of 52 studies led by Dr Natalie Molodecky and other academics from the University of Calgary, Alberta, Canada, found:

- The highest annual incidence of UC was 24.3 per 100,000 person-years in Europe, 6.3 per 100,000 person-years in Asia and the Middle East, and 19.2 per 100,000 person-years in North America.

- The highest annual incidence of CD was 12.7 per 100,000 person-years in Europe, 5.0 person-years in Asia and the Middle East, and 20.2 per 100,000 person-years in North America.

- The highest reported prevalence values for IBD were in Europe (UC, 505 per 100,000 persons; CD, 322 per 100,000 persons) and North America (UC, 249 per 100,000 persons; CD, 319 per 100,000 persons).

Note that 'incidence' refers to the number of new cases within a given time period and 'prevalence' is the proportion of cases at a specific point in time. A 'person-year' is the number of years multiplied by the numbers of people who have been affected by a certain condition.

Why is IBD increasing?

Studies in the UK have found that the number of children affected by IBD has risen by 15 per cent; in Scotland the number of childhood cases has risen by 75 per cent since 1995, according to research by the University of Edinburgh. Experts are also worried because the average age of onset of symptoms is now much earlier in childhood rather than late teens/early 20s because, as we said before, the symptoms are more severe in childhood.

Although scientists have identified a genetic basis for IBD by pinpointing many different genes, especially the variants in a gene called NOD2 in Crohn's disease – and a positive family history remains the strongest risk factor for IBD[4] – genes are clearly not the whole story. Experts refer to IBD 'as a complex genetic disorder that is influenced by environmental risk factors'.[5] Certain genes may give you a susceptibility to IBD, but the prevailing theory is that IBD is caused by a combination of genes and exposure to environmental risk factors. It's the interaction between these environmental risk factors and your normal (non-harmful) gut flora that is believed to lead to an increased immune response which results in chronic inflammation.

Possible environmental risk factors for IBD

But what are these risk factors? This has been the subject of much research over the last 30 years and scientists are unfortunately still no nearer to pinpointing the exact environmental triggers for IBD. Here's a summary of what the current thinking is.

The hygiene hypothesis

This is a popular theory – the idea that we are now 'too clean' for our own good due to improvements in sanitation and reduced exposure to infections/bacteria in childhood. Research studies have investigated the role of infections acquired in childhood to see if being exposed is protective against IBD. For example, one meta-analysis[6] (a statistical technique for combining the findings from a number of independent studies) of 23 studies found that H. pylori, an infection often acquired in childhood, was negatively associated with both Crohn's and ulcerative colitis (if you had H. pylori (see page 149) you were less likely to develop IBD). IBD is more common in developed countries where H. pylori infection is less common.

Similarly, infections with parasitic worms known collectively as helminths – such as thread worms (pin worms), hookworms and roundworms – are associated with a reduced prevalence of IBD. In one study, treating patients by infecting them with a certain type of helminth was shown to improve their symptoms compared with those given a placebo (fake treatment).[7] It's thought that helminth infections may possibly help prime the immune system in the gut against diseases that may attack in the future. Populations with good sanitation are less likely to be affected by helminths – so this fits with the hygiene hypothesis. However, a Cochrane review of two studies carried out in 2014 concluded there was insufficient evidence that helminth therapy was a safe and effective treatment and that more research was needed.[8] Cochrane reviews are systematic reviews of primary research in human health care and health policy and are internationally recognised as the highest standard in evidence-based health care. They investigate the effects of interventions for prevention, treatment and rehabilitation (see http://uk.cochrane.org/about-us for more information).

Living with multiple siblings in bigger families was also investigated as being protective against IBD – it was proposed that those who live with more siblings are exposed to more infections and that these help programme/prepare the immune system to respond to bowel infections in later life. One study found that people with Crohn's disease were shown to live in smaller families; however, similar results were not found for ulcerative colitis.[9] But other studies have found that it's the number of *older* siblings you have that's important in predicting whether you'll get IBD[10] with younger siblings most at risk.[11]

Cigarette smoking

Studies have shown smoking is implicated as a risk factor for Crohn's disease but protective against ulcerative colitis.[12] If you have Crohn's disease, smoking can increase the frequency of your flare-ups and it's more likely that you'll need surgery.[13] However, although smoking is a risk factor, the highest incidence of Crohn's disease actually occurs in countries with low rates of smoking, such as Canada.[14]

Imbalance of gut bacteria

This is an area which shows promise for more research studies. One 2011 study conducted in Belgium analysed the faecal samples of patients with Crohn's disease and compared them with their unaffected relatives and healthy controls.[15] They identified five bacterial species that characterised gut bacteria imbalance and were able to identify one type that may help restore it – raising the possibility that changing gut bacteria may have a part to play in developing future treatments for IBD.

Infections

Two infections that have been investigated as possible environmental triggers for IBD are *Salmonella* and *Campylobacter*, which both cause food poisoning symptoms. It's believed exposure to these infections may increase your risk of developing IBD.[16] A 2009 Danish study found there was a nearly threefold increase in IBD in patients who had had salmonella or campylobacter.

Diet

Diet in IBD has been an area where there has been a lot of

research. A diet rich in fruit and vegetables and high in fibre has been shown to protect against developing IBD.[17] Other studies have shown that diets high in fat, sugar, artificial sweeteners and linoleic acid found in margarines, oils and red meat[18] may put you at higher risk of IBD. Another study found that eating animal protein, including fish (but not eggs or dairy products) increased the risk of developing IBD. The Nurses' Health Study in the US found that high fibre intake recorded before the diagnosis was associated with a 30 per cent reduction in the risk of a woman developing Crohn's disease.

Experts say that many of these studies were too small to draw conclusions from and further research is still needed. It's possible though that the change in diet the industrialised world has undergone in the last 100 years, where IBD is more common, could well be one of the factors that has led to an increase in the disease.

Drugs

It's been suggested that a number of drugs may be triggers for IBD. These include the **acne drug isotretinoin** (a retinoid drug derived from vitamin A), but so far the evidence on this is inconclusive and no cause and effect relationship has been established.

Several studies have found an association between **antibiotic** use in early childhood and IBD.[19, 20] But scientists have warned against jumping to any conclusions about this as it's possible that antibiotics may have been prescribed for early undiagnosed IBD rather than triggering it.

The oral contraceptive pill has also been implicated as affecting the course of IBD and further studies have demonstrated that women with IBD who take the contraceptive pill have more flare-ups and relapses.

Non-steroidal anti-inflammatory drugs (NSAIDs) use has also been associated with risk of developing IBD in some studies.[21]

Air pollution

Studies have shown that children and young people living in areas with high levels of sulphur dioxide were at increased risk of ulcerative colitis and Crohn's disease.[22] However, other studies have highlighted that these risks may be limited to certain age groups. Hospitalisations due to IBD have also been shown to be higher in countries with high concentrations of air pollution.[23] Experts don't understand the mechanisms that may be involved, but in animal studies in laboratory conditions those exposed to air pollution have been shown to have increased levels of inflammation in the body.

Living in Northern climes/vitamin D deficiency

IBD appears to be progressively more common the further away you live from the equator (both north and south).[24] The Nurses' Health Study in the US[25] and other studies comparing populations in Northern and Southern France confirmed this. One possible explanation for this is lack of exposure to sunlight resulting in vitamin D deficiency. The body can only make vitamin D if it gets exposure to sufficiently strong sunshine (which is not available in our winters). Vitamin D is believed to have important effects on function in the immune system.

There are numerous other theories as to the triggers for IBD, but as yet none are conclusive and more research is needed. All that is established scientifically is that IBD has genetic associations, involves an abnormal reaction by the body's immune system and that this is probably triggered by something in the environment.

What are the symptoms of Crohn's disease compared to ulcerative colitis?

The short answer is that many of the symptoms overlap (around 10 per cent of IBD sufferers have a mixture of both and this is called indeterminate colitis). There are some key distinguishing characteristics your doctors will be able to tease out – see Table 6.1.

Table 6.1 Do you have Crohn's disease or ulcerative colitis?

Ulcerative colitis (just affects the colon)	Crohn's disease (can affect the whole gut)
Bloody diarrhoea and colicky abdominal pain, usually before passing a stool	Abdominal pain and diarrhoea (sometimes with blood, pus or mucus). Pain is caused when food or faeces build up after eating in an area of the intestine damaged/narrowed by inflammation
Some of or the whole colon is inflamed/ ulcerated, but other parts of the gut are usually unaffected	Patches of the gut are inflamed and ulcers may develop but there are sections that are unaffected. It mainly affects the terminal ileum (the last part of the small intestine). Sometimes Crohn's only affects the colon
Only affects the lining of the gut	Inflammation may be confined to the bowel wall but can sometimes cause deep ulcers which also penetrate deeper through the muscle layers of the bowel wall causing fistulas (an abnormal connection between one area of the body and another). Often these are around the anus. Other complications include scarring and narrowing of the intestines, sometimes leading to blockages

Ulcerative colitis (just affects the colon)	Crohn's disease (can affect the whole gut)
Inflammation is usually continuous from the rectum	Inflammation often skips segments of bowel which appear normal
Weight loss from inflammation	Weight loss from inflammation and reduced absorption
Tiredness and fatigue (anaemia is common)	Tiredness and severe fatigue (anaemia and other deficiencies occur)
Feeling feverish	Sometimes fever and night sweats can be caused by abscesses or collections of inflammation
Inflammation can involve the joints, skin, liver and eyes and cause mouth ulcers.	Inflammatory symptoms are similar to those of UC and may spread to other parts of the body causing mouth ulcers, red eyes, painful joints and rashes

Sources: Core charity and Crohn's & Colitis UK.[26, 27, 28]

More about Crohn's disease

Crohn's disease affects around one in 1,000 people and in about one in five cases if you have Crohn's disease you will have a family member who is also affected.[29]

As discussed in Table 6.1, Crohn's disease may affect any part of the gut but most commonly causes inflammation in one particular area called the terminal ileum – this is the last section of the small intestine. The first part of the colon, called the caecum, and the next, the ascending colon, are often involved. In many people only the colon is affected. Inflammation sometimes skips a segment of gut which is normal, rather than being continuous. Only a few people with Crohn's will have involvement of the stomach or the upper intestine.

Mild forms of Crohn's result in patches of inflammation – these look similar to mouth ulcers. In moderate to severe cases the intestine is damaged, and becomes thickened so it blocks the passage of digested food, causing cramp-like pain. Deep ulcers can also penetrate the bowel wall causing infection or even an abscess; this often happens around the anus. A fistula forms when an inflammatory connection goes through the skin surface, the vagina, the bladder or another part of the bowel. When inflamed tissue heals, scar tissue may form, posing a further risk of blockages in the bowel.

More about ulcerative colitis

Ulcerative colitis is the medical name for when tiny ulcers form on the surface of the lining of the large intestine. It mainly affects the rectum and lower colon, but may affect the whole of the colon. It's more common than Crohn's disease, affecting an estimated one in 420 people.[30] It seems to be more common in white people of European descent, particularly among Ashkenazi Jews who originated from Eastern Europe and Russia. It affects non-smokers and ex-smokers more than smokers, although doctors say the risks of smoking still far outweigh the possible benefits so do not take this as a licence to smoke! Men and women are affected by UC in equal numbers.

There are three types of ulcerative colitis:

- **Proctitis**. This is where only the rectum is inflamed. Fresh blood in the stools is the main symptom, plus an urgent need for the loo ('urgency') and perhaps a feeling that you have not completely emptied your bowels. You may have normal stools, diarrhoea or constipation.

- **Left sided**. This is inflammation that starts at the rectum and continues up the left side of the large intestine (the sigmoid and descending colon). Symptoms include passing diarrhoea with blood and pain on the left side of the abdomen, plus an urge to pass a stool even when your bowel is empty.

- **Total colitis.** This is sometimes called pan colitis and is when the entire colon is affected to some extent. It causes very frequent bouts of diarrhoea, severe painful stomach cramps, weight loss and often fever and generalised illness.[31]

How are Crohn's disease and ulcerative colitis diagnosed?

To be sure of a correct diagnosis your doctor will also consider other conditions with overlapping symptoms, and may undertake some or all of the following tests to rule conditions in or out as a cause of your symptoms

- **Blood tests.** A number of blood tests can reveal flags for IBD, including full blood count and other anaemia tests, checks on iron levels and sometimes ferritin (a protein that stores iron but also which increases if the body is inflamed). Important tests for other inflammatory markers will be performed such as C-reactive protein (CRP) and erythrocyte sedimentation rate (ESR). Your blood may also be tested for vitamin B12 deficiency, which is a common cause of anaemia when the ileum is inflamed in Crohn's disease. Biochemical tests, including liver function tests, will detect low levels of serum albumin, a sign of inflammation in the body, and kidney function tests can reveal if someone is dehydrated, a common side effect of diarrhoea.

- **Stool tests.** These are increasingly being used to detect the presence of IBD and look for faecal calprotectin and faecal lactoferrin proteins in particular. These proteins can be a sign of inflammation. Your doctor may also wish to exclude infections in the stool, particularly if the symptoms have been present for only a few days.

- **Biopsy.** A colonoscopy or a flexible sigmoidoscopy (see Glossary, page 180) procedure is used to take samples for a biopsy. Analyses of these samples will definitely decide if you have UC and probably decide if you have Crohn's disease. The flexible sigmoidoscopy is usually done first if colitis is suspected, as the rectum is almost always involved.

- **X-ray.** Following a barium enema (see Glossary, page 179), x-rays are taken to show the lining of your bowel.

- **CT scan.** A CT scan (see Glossary, page 181) is often performed if you are unwell with pain and fever and uses X-rays to detect abnormal areas, abscesses and many other disorders. Small-bowel Crohn's disease is often diagnosed by CT. MRI is also used. A **virtual colonoscopy** is a CT scan of your abdomen after special preparation to clear the colon (see Glossary, page 181).

- **Gastroscopy.** This procedure (see Glossary, page 183) may be used to exclude other causes of pain or anaemia and to pick up any involvement of your upper gastrointestinal tract in Crohn's.

- **Capsule endoscopy.** This procedure (see Glossary, page 182) can detect abnormal areas in the small intestine.

Treatments for Crohn's disease and ulcerative colitis

There is no drug 'cure' for IBD. A number of different types of medication are used which are designed to control or 'dampen down' inflammation in the body and control symptoms, such as diarrhoea, and help prevent complications. Patients either start on stronger drugs and step down to milder ones as control of their symptoms improves or work their way up a ladder of stronger treatments as their condition changes. Different drugs are needed to treat flare-ups and others to prevent recurrence. These include the following broad groups of drugs.

- **5-ASAs anti-inflammatories.** These are the main class of drug used to prevent relapse of colitis. Most patients with UC will have taken them and so will patients with Crohn's disease, particularly where the colon is involved. Patients with mild to moderate flare-ups of UC may take an increased dosage to control symptoms. These drugs are 5-aminosalicylates (5 ASAs), modified from aspirin, and are designed to be released in the large intestine. They include sulphasalazine, mesalazine and olsalazine. Their main use is to be prescribed long term to keep patients in remission and prevent future flare-ups. Their use has been shown to reduce the likelihood of a flare up from 85 per cent to 15 per cent in a year. They work partly by stopping white blood cells migrating to the bowel and producing inflammation in the bowel wall. They are usually well tolerated but occasionally side effects occur which include nausea/vomiting, loss of appetite, headaches and joint pain. These are more common when higher doses are taken. Rarely, kidney function can be reduced.

- **Drugs to relieve symptoms.** These include various painkillers, anti-spasmodics (including Buscopan or Mebeverine, to relieve cramping pains), laxatives (to relieve constipation) and anti-diarrhoea tablets (such as loperamide). Antibiotics, including metronidazole and ciprofloxacin, are also sometimes prescribed to treat the infections associated with IBD.

- **Corticosteroids (steroids).** These have been the mainstay of treatment to settle the initial episode and any future flares. Acute attacks of Crohn's and UC are usually treated with the steroids prednisolone and hydrocortisone. They can be given by mouth (usually as prednisolone), via injection in hospital (usually hydrocortisone) or by suppository if the patient has proctitis. They work by dampening down inflammation in the body through several different processes and are very effective as a short-term treatment to control flare-ups. They will quickly improve symptoms within days in around 80 per cent of cases.[32] They often induce a feeling of wellbeing or euphoria. Long-term use is linked with the development of unwanted effects and so prolonged use is avoided and dosages are reduced every week or so over one to two months.

  A newer drug called **budesonide** controlled release (Entocort or Budenofalk) has fewer side effects on the rest of the body but is very active in the gut and is given as tablets. Budesonide is mainly used to treat Crohn's disease of the ileum. Another steroid called **beclametasone dipropionate** (BDP or Clipper) is used to treat UC usually in combination with a 5 ASAs for a shorter time. The tablets have a coating which means they can reach the inflamed area of the gut without being dissolved in the stomach[33] and this means less of the drug enters the bloodstream and helps reduce side effects.

  As effective as steroids are in the short term, they can't prevent future flare-ups and they do have side effects which make them unsuitable for long-term use. Temporary side effects include an increase in appetite, moon face, sleep problems, facial hair growth and leg swelling. Longer-term side effects include osteoporosis, bruising more easily and diabetes. Other side effects from long-term use include mood changes, acne, moon face, increase in blood pressure / fluid retention, peptic ulcers, reduced effect of insulin, fat pad on the back, muscle wasting and osteoporosis. Because they suppress the immune system, long-term use also makes patients more susceptible to infection.

- **Immunosuppressants**. These are usually tried when steroids and 5 ASAs have failed to control UC or when steroids cannot be stopped without a relapse, particularly in Crohn's disease. As their name suggests these drugs suppress the immune system to reduce the likelihood of inflammation in the body. Commonly prescribed drugs include **azathioprine** and **mercaptopurine**. Both are used as treatments to prevent flare-ups in patients with Crohn's and UC. They take a few months to take full effect and the patient may then have to be weaned slowly off steroids after taking them. Apart from this, usually these drugs are well tolerated, safe and effective. However, a serious side effect which can occur soon after starting these medicines is bone marrow suppression leading to an infection (which has symptoms similar to 'flu), anaemia and possibly bleeding. This is usually a genetically determined individual side effect and a blood test can predict which individuals are likely to metabolise these drugs differently and so be at risk of this. Some people will need a reduced dose of the drug as a result of the predictive test. Other side effects include nausea, a sudden worsening of diarrhoea or acute pancreatitis soon after starting the drug. Possible long-term effects affecting only a few people include greater susceptibility to infections and a slightly increased risk of skin cancer and lymphoma.

Another immunosuppressant drug **methotrexate** is used in some patients with Crohn's disease who can't stop their steroid treatments without a relapse and also sometimes in patients with UC, although there's less evidence of effectiveness in these patients. Methotrexate is given once a week as a tablet or injection. It has similar side effects to other immunosuppressants and should be stopped six months before trying to become pregnant as it has been associated with birth defects. Other immunosuppressants occasionally used include **ciclosporin** and **mycophenolate mofetil** which are both used in organ transplant patients to prevent rejection. **Tacrolimus** is another treatment which can be given orally or as an ointment in severe cases of Crohn's and UC.

If you are on immunosuppressant drugs your doctors will monitor your full blood count, liver and kidney function regularly via blood tests.

- **Biologics.** These are newer drugs which are engineered to target specific elements of the immune system which are involved in inflammation and shut them down. One type of biologics agent is anti TNF – these bind to a protein produced by the body (TNF) which is a major cause of inflammation, and so helps reduce disease activity. The most commonly prescribed biologics for IBD are **infliximab** (Remicade) and **adalimumab** (Humira), but there are several others in use and in the pipeline.

Infliximab is used in cases of moderate to severe active Crohn's where immunosuppressants have not worked or have not been tolerated. It is very effective in perineal Crohn's and is sometimes used in UC as an alternative to ciclosporin. It has to be given via an infusion in hospital on an IV drip. The patent for infliximab expired in February 2015 and newer, cheaper drugs called 'biosimilars' have been launched including **Remsima** and **Inflectra**.

Adalimumab can be given every two weeks at home by the patient via an injection without the need to attend hospital and can be effective in patients in whom the benefits of infliximab have worn off. It can be difficult to decide when these drugs have had their full effect and can be stopped – often restaging (retesting to find out disease extent) is needed with CT, MRI and colonoscopy to determine how effective they have been.

Biologics have been linked to an increased risk of

infections and are usually reserved for the most severe cases when other treatments have failed. There is ongoing research investigating whether they could be more effective if used at an earlier stage of the diseases and whether this is justified given their high costs. Other side effects include joint swelling, rashes and increased risk of lymphoma. For more information on drug treatments for IBD read https://www.crohnsandcolitis.org.uk/about-inflammatory-bowel-disease/publications/drugs-used-in-ibd.

Surgery

If damage to your gut becomes extensive and your symptoms are no longer being controlled by medication your consultant may recommend surgery. In many cases this can dramatically improve your quality of life – although it's not a cure.

Surgery for ulcerative colitis

Around 20 per cent of UC patients are estimated to need surgery eventually.[34] Removing the large intestine in its entirety will stop any further inflammation in the bowel in UC. However, the remaining bowel needs to be linked up to remove faecal waste. There are two options for surgery, a proctocolectomy with permanent ileostomy, or 'pouch' surgery[35] (see Glossary, page 186).

Surgery for Crohn's disease

Around eight out of 10 patients with Crohn's may need surgery at some point.[36] You may need surgery because drugs are no longer controlling your symptoms or more commonly to remove thickened sections of your intestine, abscesses and fistulas, or rarely for bowel cancer. You're at higher risk of bowel cancer if you've had Crohn's for eight to 10 years and should be offered regular screening. Bowel cancer is more common in patients with UC who are also offered regular screening.

Some of the surgical options include a resection,[37] strictureplasty and temporary ileostomy (stoma) – see Glossary (page 184). Surgery is successful in many cases but it's important to remember it's not a cure and Crohn's can come back elsewhere.

Other treatments

- **Probiotics.** In recent years there's been tremendous interest in the concept of using bacteria in the form of probiotics (micro-organisms) to heal IBD and normalise gut function. However, a systematic review of 14 randomised controlled trials (RCTs, where an intervention group is compared with a group given a placebo) in patients with Crohn's, 21 RCTs in patients with Crohn's and five studies in patients with pouchitis (inflammation of the ileal pouch) found mixed results.[38] The review stated that in patients with Crohn's multiple studies found there was no significant difference in clinical outcomes between those who took a probiotic and those who did not and there was insufficient evidence to date to recommend them in Crohn's. However, the authors found adding a probiotic to conventional treatment improved the overall induction of and maintenance of remission in UC and there was evidence to support their use also in pouchitis.[39]

- **Faecal transplants.** Faecal microbiota transplantation (FMT) is the medical name for the infusion of a faecal suspension from a healthy person into the gastrointestinal tract of another in an attempt to treat an illness. FMT has been used successfully to treat the so-called hospital superbug *Clostridium difficile* which caused large outbreaks of severe diarrhoea in UK hospital patients in the later part of the

20th century. There are reasons to be hopeful it may also help patients with IBD, but so far the evidence is limited and mainly based on case reports. However, the authors of a systematic review, published in 2014, mentioned above concluded: 'Although limited, this evidence shows promise that FMT may be a safe but variably efficacious treatment for IBD.' They called for more RCTs to be done and for standardisation of FMT preparation, donor selection, route of administration and duration of therapy.[40] As more is learnt about the role of the microbiome in IBD, it is certain there will be further attempts to change this by FMT, but at the moment, there is no sure solution in this approach.

What about diet?

Studies don't show any one particular diet that lessens severity of symptoms or progression of the disease (although there are lots of diets out there that claim to 'cure' you). The research is contradictory at best. However, some patients do report anecdotally that they find certain foods make their symptoms worse, particularly during a flare-up (e.g. high fibre foods). Keeping a food diary can help you identify possible triggers.

Some patients are given special liquid diets during a flare-up, called **elemental or semi elemental diets**, forms of enteral nutrition which have been carefully calibrated to give them all the nutrients they need in an easily digestible form. The aim is to give the gut a chance to heal. Foods can be reintroduced gradually and this can help identify particular foods which worsen symptoms.

Many of the diets which may help IBD symptoms are actually quite hard to follow – for example the **specific carbohydrate diet**, an extreme form of a low carb diet which restricts sucrose, lactose and all grains, plus starchy foods such as parsnips and potatoes. The **low FODMAP diet** (see Chapter 3, page 37) is also very restrictive and hard to stick to in the long term.

During a flare-up your healthcare professionals may advise eating fewer fibre-rich foods to reduce the amount of insoluble fibre you are eating. Although it's healthy for most people without gut disease and adds bulk to the stools, it sits in the gut for longer and may cause bloating and pain. If you have Crohn's disease and have developed a stricture you are likely to have to be careful about the amount of insoluble fibre you eat (pips, seeds, sweetcorn, nuts, fruit and vegetable skins, the pith of fruits, beans, bran and possibly wheat). Your healthcare professional may advise you to eat white bread, white pasta and low-fibre food.

A recent article published in January 2016 by Professor James D Lewis at the University of Pennsylvania recommends patients with IBD follow a Mediterranean-style diet for its overall health benefits, but also because of its lower levels of red and processed meat and higher levels of fruit and vegetables. Professor Lewis says he also recommends his patients buy fresh food and avoid pre-packaged and processed foods.[41]

Chapter 7

Could it be cancer?

- Bowel cancer
- Stomach cancer
- Oesophageal cancer
- Gall bladder cancer
- Pancreatic cancer
- Kidney cancer
- Ovarian cancer
- Pelvic radiation disease (if you have had previous treatment for cancer)

It probably isn't cancer but...

Cancer is probably the disease that is most feared and many people choose to ignore their symptoms because they don't want to face up to having a condition that might be life-threatening – this is despite the message from the medical profession that the sooner cancer is diagnosed the greater your chances of survival. However, too many people suffer in silence until it's too late for their cancer to be cured – worrying themselves sick about what is causing their symptoms, and too scared to see a doctor.

When you suffer from stomach pains, changes in bowel habit, persistent acid reflux, or bloating, cancer is *least* likely to be the cause, but you should still see your doctor to have it ruled out. This is particularly important if your symptoms have coincided with other vaguer symptoms including unexplained weight loss and/or fatigue, which could be due to anaemia. Blood in your stools is far more likely to be caused by piles (haemorrhoids), but many of the symptoms can be similar. Likewise, bloating is far more likely to be due to IBS than ovarian cancer and intense pain in your gall bladder is more likely to be caused by gallstones than gall bladder cancer.

Equally though, you are not qualified to make these distinctions – you need to tell your doctor about them so he or she can investigate them and rule out anything life-threatening. Your doctor will recognise certain 'red flag' symptoms (see Chapter 2, page 18) and make an urgent referral to rule out cancer if necessary.

The good news about cancer

The good news is that survival rates for many cancers have improved dramatically: UK bowel cancer survival rates for instance have doubled in the past 40 years[1] and now have a 60 per cent 10-year survival rate.[2] The earlier the cancer is detected the higher the survival rate; for example, men with stage 2 bowel cancer have an 80 per cent five-year survival rate and women a 90 per cent five-year survival rate. This compares with a five-year survival rate of only 5 per cent in men and 10 per cent in women if the cancer has already reached stage 4 and spread beyond the bowel, according to figures from Cancer Research UK.[3]

The worst case scenario could be that your symptoms are of cancer, but even if that does turn out to be the case, the earlier you are diagnosed and treated the better -- so don't ignore your symptoms.

Sometimes it's possible your GP might mistake your gut symptoms for a non-life-threatening condition such as IBS – but there are usually red flag symptoms that will ring alarm bells with them, and encourage them to investigate your symptoms more and refer you on to a specialist. Make sure they know about any cancers that have occurred at an early age in your family. If you're not happy with your GP's diagnosis and your symptoms are having a big impact on your quality of life, keep going back – take a symptom diary with you and ask to be referred to a gastroenterologist or seek a second opinion.

Bowel cancer

Bowel cancer (also known as colorectal cancer) is the fourth most common cancer overall in the UK, with 41,600 cases diagnosed every year – around 110 people a day. Incidence of colorectal cancer increased in 27 of 51 countries between 1983 and 2002.[4] This is predicted to rise from 1.4 million new cases worldwide in 2012 to 2.4 million cases by 2035 as more countries adopt a Western lifestyle, characterised by obesity, high meat consumption, lack of physical activity, low levels of fruit and vegetable consumption, smoking and high alcohol intake.[5] Throughout Europe it's the second most common cancer with 447,000 cases diagnosed in 2012.

In the UK, bowel cancer is the second biggest cancer killer, causing one death every 30 minutes according to the charity Beating Bowel Cancer.[6] But it is also curable and easily diagnosed.

Symptoms of bowel cancer

The symptoms of bowel cancer unfortunately overlap with other less serious medical complaints, including piles (haemorrhoids) (see Chapter 9, page 168), so the symptoms can either be wrongly dismissed, or cause worry and anxiety when all that is needed is a change in diet and some haemorrhoid cream. The trouble is it can be difficult to tell them apart yourself, so ask your GP if you need a rectal examination or further tests. In other words, you have to be vigilant in looking out for changes in your bowel habit but equally be aware that it probably isn't down to cancer.

Symptoms include:
- Bleeding from your back passage (blood in your poo)
- A feeling of having to strain in your back passage even after you have passed a stool (also called incomplete evacuation)
- A change in your bowel habits (going more frequently, or less often, runny or harder stool)
- A lump you can feel in your abdomen (most commonly on the right) or in your rectum
- Unexplained weight loss
- Pain in your abdomen
- Anaemia (due to low red blood cell count) – related symptoms can include tiredness and breathlessness.

Most cases of bowel cancer are in the over 50 age group – around 90 per cent - so if you're experiencing any of the above symptoms and are under 50 it's highly unlikely to be bowel cancer. Bright red blood in your stools is most likely piles (see page 168) – swollen veins which can be damaged by straining to pass a bowel movement. Blood mixed in with the stools, which may be darker red blood or tar like, could occasionally be a sign of cancer higher up the bowel.

Having said that, cases of bowel cancer are on the increase in the under 50s,[7] so don't be complacent. It is particularly important to let your doctor know if you have any family history of bowel cancer or polyps, as your chances are higher if you have a first degree relative (mother, father, siblings) who has had bowel cancer. There are good recommendations regarding when you should have tests like a colonoscopy to detect any cancer when it is early and easily treated.

Other conditions which can increase your risk include having inflammatory bowel disease (see Chapter 6, page 95) or having previous polyps removed.[8]

How is bowel cancer diagnosed?

If you go and see your GP complaining of blood in your stools he or she may perform a rectal examination with a gloved finger to check for swelling or lumps in your rectum and for haemorrhoids. They may also run a blood test to check for anaemia, another symptom of bowel cancer, and additionally perform a stool test to detect inflammation (faecal calprotectin).

If you are referred on to a specialist, they will take a detailed medical history from you and order further investigations. These could include a flexible sigmoidoscopy and/or a colonoscopy (see Glossary, page 181).

- **Flexible sigmoidoscopy.** Doctors use this procedure to get a good look at the lining of the rectum and the lower part of the large bowel and can take biopsies of any suspicious areas. It's estimated that some bowel cancers can take between five and 10 years to develop and may start as a non-cancerous small growth called a polyp. These polyps may turn cancerous later on, when they can grow into the muscle layers behind the lining of the bowel, but they can easily be removed. If one polyp is found, then the entire colon should be checked by a colonoscopy.

- **Colonoscopy.** If polyps are found during this procedure they can be removed using a wire loop.

What are the treatment options for bowel cancer?

Polyps are easily taken out at colonoscopy and this will prevent the ones that have been found changing into cancer. Other new polyps usually take several years to develop and further colonoscopies are usually planned when polyps have been removed, particularly if they are multiple.

If either the biopsy samples, or the polyps removed, are found to be cancerous you will then be cared for by a multi-disciplinary team including surgeons and cancer specialists. You will probably get CT or other scans to find out the stage your cancer has reached when diagnosed. The treatment options include surgery to remove the cancer (if possible) through a procedure called a colectomy (see Glossary, page 180). If the cancer is advanced, doctors may still be able to slow its progress by using chemotherapy and radiotherapy to shrink the tumours, and sometimes this is done before later surgery.

How can I lower my risk of bowel cancer?

- **Change your lifestyle.** In 2012, the Word Cancer Research Fund Institute estimated 47 per cent of cases of colorectal cancer cases could be prevented by eating and drinking healthily. The WCRF's Continuous Update Project said there was convincing evidence that eating red meat and processed meat, drinking alcohol, body fatness and abdominal fatness all increased the risk of colorectal cancer. In the UK the Department of Health advises eating no more than 70 g a day of red meat (lamb, beef, pork etc.). Reducing processed meats that have been cured or smoked, including bacon, sausages, salami etc., is also important to reduce the risk of bowel cancer.[9,10] Other advice on prevention is to keep to a healthy weight, stop smoking, avoid drinking too much alcohol, take care to get the 150 minutes per day of brisk exercise and to eat more fibre-rich foods, such as cereals and pulses.

- **Take part in national bowel cancer screening programmes.** Regular screening has been shown to cut the risk of dying from bowel cancer by 16 per cent.[11] In some parts of the UK a flexible sigmoidoscopy (see Glossary, page 183) is offered to people around their 55th birthday as part of a national pilot scheme which is currently being evaluated. Additionally, home test kits for faecal occult blood (FOB) in stools are sent out to people aged 60 to 74 every two years. They collect stool samples to wipe on a special card and then send them to a laboratory in a special, hygienically-sealed envelope. Around 98 out of 100 people will get a normal result, but the remainder may need the test to be repeated and others may be called for a colonoscopy.[12]

- **Report any new symptoms promptly** especially if you have a new change in bowel habits, and get tested.

- **Know your family risk.** If you have been unlucky and there is bowel cancer in your family, be sure you know what tests are recommended and when you should have them.

Stomach cancer

There are around 7,300 cases of stomach cancer diagnosed every year in the UK. The big problem with it is that early symptoms, which can include persistent heartburn and indigestion, trapped wind, and frequent burping, are obviously easily confused with other common digestive complaints, such as stomach ulcers, and this means that it is very often not diagnosed until a late stage. Because of late diagnosis five-year survival rates are relatively low when compared with breast or bowel cancer, with 41.8 per cent surviving a year, 18.9 per cent five years and 15 per cent 10 years.[13] However, the figures need careful interpretation as they reflect the fact that most cancers are diagnosed at a late stage; latest figures from the American Cancer Society in 2015[14] show that stomach cancer diagnosed before it has spread outside the stomach has a five-year survival rate of 64 per cent. Getting diagnosed early is therefore very important.

Later symptoms of stomach cancers include weight loss, anaemia, loss of appetite, lumpiness and swelling in the stomach due to fluid build-up, vomiting of food, difficulty swallowing, and yellowing of the skin and the whites of your eyes.

If any of the above symptoms are new and you're in your 40s or over, go and see your doctor. As we've said earlier, the chances are they are not caused by cancer but it's better to be on the safe side.

What are the risk factors for stomach cancer?

- **Age.** The majority of people diagnosed with stomach cancer in the UK are aged 55 or over and the average age of diagnosis is 70.

- **Smoking.** Smokers are twice as likely to develop stomach cancer as non-smokers and 20 per cent of all stomach cancer cases are in smokers.

- *Helicobacter pylori.* This is a common bacterial infection which lives in the gut in around 40 per cent of people in the UK (about 50 per cent worldwide).[15] In most people it causes no problems at all, but in about 15 per cent it can attack the lining of the stomach causing recurrent indigestion, and, over time, ulcers in the stomach and the duodenum may develop (see Chapter 8, page 139). This can be dangerous if they perforate or start to bleed. It can be treated with antibiotics. *H. pylori* infection not only produces symptoms which can seem like cancer, but it is also associated with a higher risk of developing stomach cancer, so if someone in the family has had stomach cancer it may be worth your being tested and treated for *H. pylori* if the bacteria is found, to reduce your risk. More research is ongoing to see if this reduces cancer risk.

- **Diet high in pickles/salt.** Eating a diet high in pickled fish and vegetables, which contain nitrates, a preservative, increases the risk of stomach cancer. One meta-analysis published in 2012 found a potential 50 per cent higher risk of gastric cancer associated with pickled vegetables and other foods and perhaps an even stronger association in countries such as Korea and China where high volumes of pickled food are consumed.[16]

- **Genes.** In about one in 50 cases of stomach cancer a gene mutation called E-cadherin is involved, but in most cases there is no family history of the disease, so genetic screening is not usually offered.

Diagnosis of stomach cancer

Stomach cancer is usually diagnosed by a gastroscopy, or a CT or MRI scan (see Glossary).

Treatment

If the cancer hasn't advanced to other parts of the body, it can be removed by taking out all or part of the stomach. If the cancer has spread, chemotherapy and radiotherapy may be used to shrink the tumour and slow down its progress.

Oesophageal cancer

Cancer of the oesophagus, the tube which carries food and water from the mouth to the stomach (sometimes called the gullet), is diagnosed in 8,300 people every year in the UK, making it the 13th most common cancer. Worldwide, it is the eighth most common cancer and the sixth most common cause of cancer death.[17] Its incidence has been increasing worldwide over the past decade.[18] Men are twice as likely as women to develop it.[19]

The key symptoms include difficulties swallowing (known as dysphagia), pain or a burning sensation when you swallow, or a sensation of food sticking in your throat. Other symptoms can include weight loss (because you are not swallowing enough food), persistent indigestion, a persistent cough, hoarseness, vomiting and coughing up blood.

Risk and prevention

Experts say the majority of oesophageal cancer cases could be prevented by a healthy lifestyle. You're at higher risk of oesophageal cancer if you:

- **Smoke and drink a lot of alcohol.** These are the two main risk factors – and doing both is definitely worse, because drinking alcohol makes it easier for harmful chemicals from smoking to be absorbed in the mouth and throat. One study found that people who drank up to five units of alcohol and smoked eight cigarettes a day increased their risk of oesophageal cancer by between 13 (for men) and 19 times (for women).[20]

- **GORD.** You are at higher risk if you have a history of gastro-oesophageal reflux disease (GORD). This is where stomach acid travels up into the oesophagus because a valve between the stomach and oesophagus becomes weak and relaxes. This irritates the lining of the oesophagus causing a burning sensation and inflammation in the throat.

- **Barrett's oesophagus.** Experts say that one in 11 people with chronic acid reflux will develop Barrett's oesophagus.[21, 22] This condition can cause abnormal cells to develop in the lining of the oesophagus and one study says it increases the risk of oesophageal cancer developing between 50 and 100 times.[23]

- **Age.** Eighty per cent of oesophageal cancer cases are in the over 60s.

- **Being overweight/obese.** A Cancer Research UK study estimated that being overweight or obese caused more than 25 per cent of oesophageal cancers in men and more than one in 10 in women. The most likely explanation for this is that overweight people are more likely to suffer from acid reflux and this may lead to Barrett's oesophagus, a risk factor for cancer (see above).[24]

- **Drinking hot drinks.** A 2009 review of 59 studies published in the *International Journal of Cancer* concluded[25] that 'the results strongly suggest that high-temperature beverage drinking increased the risk of oesophageal cancer'. Experts believe it's possible that very hot drinks may cause thermal damage to cells lining the oesophagus.

- **Poor diet.** Low fruit and vegetable intake is also a risk factor. Cancer Research UK estimates that four out of 10 cases of oesophageal cancer could be prevented if people ate five portions or more of fruit and vegetables every day.[26]

Diagnosis and treatment of oesophageal cancer

If you've been previously diagnosed with Barrett's oesophagus, your condition may have been regularly monitored by a specialist so if cancer does develop it's likely to be detected at an earlier stage. You should have been offered regular endoscopies to check for cancerous cells in your oesophagus.

Cancer of the oesophagus is usually diagnosed by endoscopy and biopsies, or X-rays after a barium swallow (see Glossary, page 179).

NICE has produced new guidelines for referral for investigations for upper GI cancers in 2015.[28] The guidelines say patients who have difficulty swallowing and weight loss and one of either dyspepsia, reflux or abdominal pain, should be referred for urgent gastrointestinal endoscopy within two weeks.

Treatment options depend on the stage the cancer has reached and include surgery to remove the cancer, chemotherapy and radiotherapy.

As we said before, the number of patients who survive one year or more is 40 per cent, 15 per cent for five years and 10 per cent at 10 years.[28] This reflects the fact that so many oesophageal cancers have been diagnosed at a late stage. New data from an audit conducted in 2014 found that 40 per cent of oesophageal cancer patients are able to have treatment to cure their cancer but it is important to diagnose this early.[29]

Gall bladder cancer

Gall bladder cancer is rare, but there were 1,923 cases diagnosed in 2013 in the UK. The gall bladder is a pear-shaped organ that is found under the liver and its job is to store bile, a liquid produced by the liver to reduce fat.

Seventy per cent of gall bladder cancer cases are in women and it's much more common in the elderly. Other risk factors include being overweight and having had gall stones (see Chapter 8, page 152) in the past, or another condition called cholecystitis (swelling and inflammation of the gall bladder (see Chapter 8, page 156) as well as diabetes.

Unfortunately, there aren't any early symptoms but later ones can include feeling sick, abdominal pain (particularly in the upper right portion of the abdomen) and yellow skin and yellow sclera (whites of the eyes). Others include a swollen stomach and unexplained weight loss, itching and fever.[30]

It can be diagnosed via a number of investigations, including ultrasound, ERCP (an X-ray using an endoscope), CT or MRI looking at the gall bladder. Treatment options include surgery – ranging from removal of the gall bladder to more radical surgery where lymph nodes and surrounding organs such as the pancreas and duodenum are also removed. Chemotherapy and radiotherapy may also be needed.[31]

The fact that gall bladder cancer is often diagnosed late means that the outlook can be poor. No national statistics are available in the UK, but Cancer Research UK estimates five-year survival is around 10 per cent, based on evidence from clinical papers.

The World Cancer Research Fund advises one in six cases could be prevented by keeping to a healthy weight. [32]

Pancreatic cancer

The pancreas is a gland which produces enzymes needed to digest food, and hormones, including insulin, which regulates blood sugar. It's tucked away, deep inside the abdomen behind the stomach which is part of the reason why pancreatic cancer tends to be diagnosed late as it doesn't have any visible swelling or lumps in the early stages.

Symptoms of pancreatic cancer tend to come at a later stage and can include pain in the back or upper abdomen, unexpected weight loss and jaundice (yellow skin tone and yellowing of the whites of the eyes – although this is more likely to be caused by gallstones (see Chapter 8, page 152). Another possible symptom recently recognised is the onset of type 1 diabetes in people who are not overweight. The pain tends to come and go and is worse when lying down or after eating. Other symptoms include itching (caused by jaundice), indigestion, changes in bowel habits (particularly pale, fatty, foul-smelling stools)[33] and fevers with shivering.

Pancreatic cancer is high profile these days because there has been much campaigning and lobbying by cancer charities for greater awareness and more funding for research into new treatments. The deaths of Apple boss Steve Jobs, actor Patrick Swayze and opera singer Luciano Pavarotti have made pancreatic cancer more talked about, but survival rates remain low. The unexpected survival of the rock guitarist Wilko Johnson shows how the rare form of pancreatic neuroendocrine tumour (NET) has a much better prognosis.

There are currently around 8,800 cases of pancreatic cancer in the UK every year. Sadly, one-year survival is just 20 per cent and the figure is 5 per cent for five years or more, and one per cent survive 10 years or more.[34] Some doctors report higher survival rates on clinical trials though, and newer treatments have recently become available which may extend life.

New referral guidelines from NICE published in 2015[35]

recommend GPs refer anyone over 40 with jaundice for an urgent CT scan and also people over 60 who have weight loss, diarrhoea, back pain, abdominal pain, vomiting, constipation and new onset of diabetes. It is hoped that more prompt investigations may improve the outlook for pancreatic cancer patients. New blood and urine tests are also being developed in a bid to detect more early stage cancers.[36, 37] There have also been some breakthroughs in investigating new treatments for the disease.[38]

Current treatment options may include surgery – but only up to one in five patients is suitable for curative surgery as the cancer has usually spread by the time it is diagnosed. The surgical options can include removal of the head of the pancreas, duodenum, gall bladder and bile duct, or the Whipple procedure (named after Allen Whipple who first performed the operation), where all of the former are removed plus part of the stomach; there is a third operation where the whole pancreas is removed.

Chemotherapy may also be given after surgery or in combination with radiotherapy.

Kidney cancer

There are around 10,144 new cases of kidney cancer diagnosed every year in the UK and 4,252 deaths. The good news is that survival has greatly improved, up from 25 per cent five-year survival in the 1970s to 50 per cent in 2012.[39]

The most common symptom is blood in your urine (this might not be visible though and only detectable in a urine test), as well as a lump in the kidney area. Other symptoms are vaguer but include a pain in the side below the ribs that doesn't go away, tiredness and weight loss and sometimes a high temperature, high blood pressure and anaemia.

Kidney cancer can be diagnosed by a number of tests, including a urine test to check for blood in the urine (there are many other causes of blood in the urine, though most of them not serious), or a CT urogram (see Glossary).

Risk factors for kidney cancer are largely lifestyle-related – around 42 per cent are thought to be preventable, with smoking and being overweight being the most significant risk factors. However, there are some risk factors you can't do anything about, such as age (it's more common as you get older) and your height (being very tall puts you more at risk).[40]

Treatment options include surgery to remove the affected kidney plus chemotherapy and radiotherapy.

Ovarian cancer

Ovarian cancer obviously isn't a cancer of the gut but the symptoms can involve the gut and include bloating, feeling full or abdominal pain, and these are easy to dismiss as IBS in the early stages. Such symptoms may include a swollen tummy, feeling bloated all the time, tummy and pelvic pain, needing to wee more often, feeling full very quickly when eating, or pain during intercourse.[41] The cancer charity Target Ovarian Cancer says the key things to remember are that the symptoms will be 'persistent, frequent and new'.[42]

Ovarian cancer is most common in women who have gone through their menopause and affects 7,100 women a year in the UK. Only a small proportion (10 per cent) of cases are linked to genetic factors, such as the BRAC1 and BRAC2 genes, which are also associated with breast cancer. The main risk factors appear to be increasing age, being overweight and smoking. Other factors include hormonal changes – breastfeeding, pregnancy and taking the contraceptive pill are reported to be protective against ovarian cancer.[43]

According to Cancer Research UK, one-year survival for ovarian cancer in England and Wales is 73 per cent; 46 per cent of women survive five years or more and 35 per cent survive 10 years or more. If you are diagnosed at stage 1, the outlook is much better with a 90 per cent five-year survival rate, compared with only 5 per cent at stage 4.

If your GP suspects ovarian cancer, he or she can order a blood screening test for a biomarker called CA125 – raised levels can indicate ovarian cancer in 50 per cent of women with early stages of ovarian cancer. If you've got new irritable bowel-type symptoms and are aged over 50, it's also a good idea to get your CA125 levels checked. You may also be referred for ultrasound scans and if a suspected mass is found, you may have a procedure called fine needle aspiration (see Glossary, page 183).

Treatment options include surgery or a combination of surgery and chemotherapy.

Pelvic radiation disease

There are currently two million people in the UK who are cancer survivors (defined as living with and beyond cancer) and this number has been predicted to increase to four million by 2030.[44] Whilst it's obviously good news that so many people now survive cancer in the long term, the downside is that there is now a new generation of patients who have to live with the long-term side effects of surgery, chemotherapy and radiotherapy. These effects commonly involve the gut.

Sometimes patients who've had radiation treatment for cancer in the pelvic area develop bowel and bladder symptoms associated with radiation damage. This is known as pelvic radiation disease (PRD) and affects around 17,000 new patients a year in the UK. This is more than the number of new patients with inflammatory bowel diseases, yet few people have heard of the condition. Reports show how PRD can cause any of 22 different gastrointestinal symptoms,[45] simultaneously in some cases, and can adversely affect quality of life, making some people effectively housebound unless they get treatment. One of the problems is that the symptoms often start long after the treatment has finished so patients may not realise they are connected to their radiotherapy and may also no longer be under the care of an oncology team. As a result, many suffer in silence and never get appropriate help.

According to the Pelvic Radiation Disease Association (see page 136*), the symptoms can include:

- Needing the toilet urgently
- Feeling you haven't emptied your bowel
- Needing to go more frequently
- Bloating and noisy rumblings in your tummy
- Excess or smelly gas/burping
- Diarrhoea, loose and smelly, fatty stools
- Constipation
- Waking at night to pass a stool
- Bleeding from the bottom
- Leaking from the bottom/mucus from the bottom
- Soiling underwear
- Tummy pain, cramps
- Trouble holding in wind
- Struggling to pass stools
- Losing control of your bowel
- Having to wear incontinence pads in case of accidents[46]
- Diarrhoea caused by small intestinal bacterial overgrowth (SIBO, see Chapter 5, page 92).

Other associations include bile acid malabsorption (see Chapter 5, page 79), which may cause frequent watery diarrhoea.[47]

The important thing to remember is that these symptoms can develop many months after treatment has ended so it might not be immediately apparent that they are connected to your cancer treatment.

Radiotherapy also causes changes in other pelvic organs and patients may also notice bladder problems, including needing to pass urine more frequently, incontinence, urgency, experiencing a burning sensation while passing urine, and bleeding and loss of sex drive in women and erection problems in men.

Getting treatment for pelvic radiation disease

It is easier to get treatment if you are still being seen by your cancer specialist and team; mention pelvic radiation disease symptoms to them, and they can either offer medication and lifestyle advice, or refer you to a gastroenterologist for other more specialist treatments. But some of the symptoms can develop much later when you are no longer under the care of your cancer team, and it can be harder to get the right help. Patients who do not receive expert care locally or regionally should ask to be referred by their GP or specialist to one of the centres with expertise in this condition. The Pelvic Radiation Disease Association can offer help and advice about referrals to specialists in PRD.

It is not the case that patients just have to put up with PRD symptoms. Many treatments are available including: drugs, dietary advice, biofeedback, pelvic floor exercises, toileting exercises and perhaps antibiotic treatment. Recognising the condition and getting a clear diagnosis as to what is going on is most of the issue. More specialist treatments may include hyperbaric oxygen therapy, where patients breathe in oxygen at higher concentrations than atmospheric pressure in a chamber. This causes oxygen to be absorbed by all cells and tissues in the body, even those with reduced blood flow, and this can help restore function to damaged tissue. This is only available in selected NHS centres around the UK. However, gastroenterologists should be able to offer treatment for most of the other symptoms if they are correctly diagnosed.

* The checklist on page 134 is reproduced by permission of the Pelvic Radiation Disease Society www.pdra.org.uk. Telephone +44 (0) 1372 744388.

Chapter 8

Is it 'just' indigestion?

Symptom checker

If you have one or more of the following symptoms, you may have one of the conditions discussed in this chapter.

- Burning sensation, fullness, heaviness or ache in upper abdomen or lower chest
- Burning, griping pain in the abdomen, lower gut and back
- Sharp, persistent pain at the top of the stomach or above ribs on right
- Bitter taste in the mouth
- Nausea, vomiting
- Bloating
- Belching and burping
- Lump in your throat
- Tickly cough

Indigestion

Indigestion is that uncomfortable feeling most of us have experienced at some point in the upper abdomen or lower part of the chest – usually after eating or drinking (but not always).

The official medical definition is upper abdominal discomfort or pain that may be described as a burning sensation, heaviness or an ache. It is often related to eating and may be accompanied by other symptoms, such as nausea, fullness in the upper abdomen or belching.[1] It's usually worse if you lie down directly after eating a heavy meal. Other names for it include dyspepsia and acid reflux or heartburn. It is basically an inflammation of the gullet (oesophagus) – the long pipe that runs from the mouth to the stomach.

Indigestion is so common most people will have experienced it at some time and it's usually more of a fleeting inconvenience than a major health problem. Most people don't see their doctor about it and either grin and bear it or simply treat it themselves with remedies they can buy over the counter from a chemist. Only a quarter of people who suffer indigestion see their GP about their symptoms and about 10 per cent of these consultations will be referred for further investigations.[2]

Indigestion is rarely a symptom of a serious underlying medical condition (but if you are worried, see Box 8.1). In people who have an endoscopy (see Glossary, page 181) to investigate their indigestion, 30 per cent will have no abnormal findings and 10 to 17 per cent will have oesophagitis (inflammation of the oesophagus) and the rest will have gastric or duodenal ulcers, gastritis, duodenitis (inflammation of the duodenum) or hiatus hernias, according to the British Society of Gastroenterology.[3] But, having said that, we're not saying indigestion can't still affect your quality of life and be a pain to deal with.

If you've bought this book, it may be that you're one of the unfortunate ones who suffer from recurrent severe bouts of indigestion. We're hoping this chapter may help you get to the root of what's causing your symptoms, help you find some long-term relief and enable you to enjoy your food again.

What causes indigestion?

Diet

Most people associate indigestion with overdoing it, with a big meal, sometimes with a high fat or spice content – creamy curry sauces and dishes containing chilli for instance. You might also notice that particular foods can trigger your symptoms, including curries, fatty foods, citrus fruits, bananas and cucumbers – it's very individual though. Sometimes however, it can be down to something simple such as eating too fast or too close to bedtime. Drinking too much alcohol, or caffeine in coffee, tea and chocolate may have a similar effect.

Drug side effects

But there are many other causes of indigestion and sometimes the cause isn't so obvious. These other causes include the **side effects of drugs**, including non-steroidal anti-inflammatory drugs (NSAIDs) taken to relieve the pain of arthritis (such as ibuprofen and aspirin) and nitrates prescribed for angina for instance.

Acid reflux or GORD

But a major cause of recurring indigestion is acid reflux, or **gastro-oesophageal reflux disease (GORD)**, which is caused by the sphincter in the oesophagus failing to close and prevent large amounts of stomach contents, including acid, moving back up from the stomach and causing irritation and inflammation in the oesophagus. The inside of the oesophagus has a protective lining but it can become irritated and inflamed by stomach acid. If the lining becomes ulcerated by the stomach acid, it causes a condition called **oesophagitis**.

Sometimes stomach acid can escape back up from the stomach to the oesophagus due to **gastric and duodenal ulcers** (known collectively as **peptic ulcers**), which are sores which develop in the lining of the stomach or duodenum. Peptic ulcers can be caused by a bacterial infection called *Helicobacter pylori*.

Another cause of GORD is **hiatus hernia** – where part of the stomach pushes up through the diaphragm (the sheet of muscle between the abdomen and the chest, needed for breathing), partially blocking refluxed stomach acid in the oesophagus.

Being overweight or obese (including weight gain due to pregnancy) will make it more likely you'll suffer from acid reflux – obesity causes more pressure in the abdomen which forces acid back up into the gullet. This is also true if you are constipated or wearing clothes with a tight waistband. Chemicals in cigarette smoke can also relax the ring of muscle that divides the stomach from the oesophagus and make it easier for stomach acid to escape back into the gullet, causing acid reflux/heartburn symptoms. Stress and anxiety are also believed to play a part in indigestion, as is increasing age.

If you have some of the 'alarm bell' symptoms described in Box 8.1 you should be considered for urgent endoscopy referral rather than taking any prolonged treatments which may mask the symptoms of a more serious illness.

Box 8.1 Reasons for an urgent referral

NICE advises that:[4]
- people with an upper abdominal mass require **urgent referral** for endoscopic investigation (an appointment within two weeks) [National Collaborating Centre for Cancer, 2015].
- **urgent direct access** upper gastrointestinal endoscopy should be performed within two weeks to assess for stomach cancer in people with dysphagia

---

> (swallowing problems) or aged 55 and over with weight loss and any of the following: upper abdominal pain, reflux, dyspepsia.
>
> - referral for **non-urgent direct access upper gastrointestinal endoscopy** should be considered to assess for stomach cancer in people with haematemesis (vomiting blood) and in people aged 55 or over with treatment-resistant dyspepsia, upper abdominal pain with low haemoglobin levels, or raised platelet count with any of the following: nausea, vomiting, weight loss, reflux, dyspepsia, upper abdominal pain; or nausea or vomiting with any of the following: weight loss, reflux, dyspepsia, upper abdominal pain [National Collaborating Centre for Cancer, 2015].

More about GORD and how it's treated

In gastro-oesophageal reflux disease (GORD), gastric contents (bile, acid and food) leak up from the stomach into the oesophagus causing symptoms such as heartburn and acid regurgitation into the mouth. This is because a ring of muscle called the lower oesophageal sphincter muscle (LOS), which acts as a valve at the bottom of the oesophagus (gullet), weakens. Normally the LOS muscle opens to allow food to enter the stomach, but in GORD it allows stomach acid to leak out of the stomach into the oesophagus where it causes acid reflux (stomach acid comes back up from the stomach into your throat and mouth, causing an unpleasant taste), heartburn (a burning sensation behind the breastbone) or problems with swallowing, due to a narrowing of the oesophagus. Other symptoms can include a persistent cough which is worse at night, nausea, chest pain, tiredness and wheezing. Asthmatics may also find that their asthma symptoms are aggravated by GORD.[5]

GORD is one of the main causes of recurrent indigestion. When it's defined as one or more episodes of heartburn and/acid regurgitation, prevalence in the Western world ranges between 10 and 20 per cent of the population.[6] You're more at risk of GORD if you're overweight, eat large amounts of fatty food (as fatty foods delay gastric emptying) and drink too much caffeine (including coffee, tea or chocolate), smoke, or drink too much alcohol – as all of these lifestyle factors are believed to reduce the muscle tone of the LOS muscle. It's also more common in pregnancy when rising levels of the hormones progesterone and oestrogen can weaken the LOS. Side effects of certain medicines, including calcium channel blockers used to treat high blood pressure, nitrates prescribed for angina and benzodiazepines for anxiety, can also increase the symptoms of GORD. It is common in people who have a hiatus hernia (see page 145).

Most people are able to manage their symptoms themselves by making some lifestyle changes, including losing weight, eating smaller, more frequent meals, avoiding particular foods, eating earlier in the evening (at least three to four hours before bedtime), sleeping on their left side or by raising the head of their bed by four to eight inches (10 to 20 cm) by placing bricks or solid wood under it (don't prop yourself up with pillows as this can increase abdominal pressure and make the problem worse), avoiding too much alcohol or caffeine, stopping smoking and cutting down on rich, fatty and spicy foods. Learning to manage stress, anxiety and depression may also be helpful, as there's some evidence that people who suffer from these conditions are more likely to suffer from GORD.

Over-the-counter remedies can be used to treat mild to moderate cases of GORD. The most popular pills and liquid medicines include antacids to neutralise the effects of stomach acid and alginates which coat the lining of the oesophagus and the stomach to protect them from stomach acid. However, although antacids and alginates are commonly bought and prescribed for GORD, and they relieve symptoms rapidly, there isn't much evidence of their long-term effectiveness for GORD.[7] The recommended first-line medical treatment in the UK is lifestyle advice, plus a one-month course of drugs called proton pump inhibitors (PPIs) (for example, omeprazole, esomeprazole, pantoprazole, rabeprazole or lansoprazole). These drugs reduce the amount of stomach acid produced and are now very widely prescribed: 57.7 million items were prescribed in England and Wales for dyspepsia, GORD and to prevent ulcers from NSAI drugs according to data published in 2015 – a 135 per cent increase in 10 years.

However, one review found that between 10 and 40 per cent of people with GORD who are prescribed PPIs fail to experience an improvement in their symptoms on standard dose PPIs.[8] If your symptoms persist it is important to go back to your doctor as they may need to increase the dose and/or prescribe PPIs for another month. Sometimes taking the PPI twice daily or just with your evening meal will be effective for night-time symptoms.

Your doctor may also want to add or substitute another drug called an H2 receptor antagonist, particularly if you have night-time symptoms that have not responded to PPIs. These work by blocking the effects of a chemical called histamine, which is needed to produce stomach acid. H2 blockers include ranitidine, cimetidine, famotidine and nizatidine.

Unfortunately, the lifestyle changes (especially weight loss) which are recommended are hard to achieve for many people and GORD symptoms have been shown to recur in 80 per cent of cases within a year. Doctors are advised to attempt to discontinue PPIs and other medication use after two months to avoid unnecessary prescribing costs. However, in many cases long-term prescription of PPIs is needed – at the lowest dose that can effectively control symptoms.

Some low dose versions of H2 blockers are available over the counter and higher doses on prescription.

If your symptoms haven't improved after two months of PPIs, the National Institute for Health and Care Excellence (NICE) recommends that your doctor considers referring you for further investigations and management.

Long-term complications of GORD

If GORD symptoms are severe and long term then complications can develop. These include:

*   **Oesophagitis and oesophageal ulcers.** Inflammation of the lining of the oesophagus (oesophagitis) can develop, leading to redness and soreness. Over time this can lead to oesophageal ulcers – painful sores in the oesophagus which can bleed and make swallowing painful. These can be treated by PPIs to address the underlying cause of GORD.

*   **Oesophageal strictures.** This is where scar tissue forms due to repeated damage to the lining of the oesophagus and makes swallowing food painful and difficult. The stricture can be treated by inserting an endoscopy tube into the oesophagus and inflating a tiny balloon to enlarge the space. This procedure can be performed under local anaesthetic.

*   **Barrett's oesophagus.** Long-term GORD can be associated with abnormal or pre-cancerous changes in the cells lining the oesophagus, called Barrett's oesophagus. It is estimated around 10 per cent of people with GORD will have this condition.[8A] Most cases develop in the 50 to 70 age group.[9]

Most people have no symptoms at all but in those that do, heartburn and indigestion are the most common ones. Other symptoms include feeling sick, vomiting and problems swallowing food, and more unusually, vomiting blood.

Barrett's oesophagus is diagnosed via an endoscopy (see Glossary) where appearances on inspecting the lower end of the oesophagus show an irregular boundary with the stomach lining. Biopsies are taken to check for any pre-cancerous changes. If you are diagnosed with Barrett's oesophagus you may be advised to have regular endoscopies to check for the development of any new pre-cancerous changes. We should stress though that only a small number of people with Barrett's oesophagus go on to develop oesophageal cancer (see Chapter 7, page 126).

Treatment options include all those listed on page 126, including lifestyle changes and PPIs to reduce acid. Most people with Barrett's oesophagus will need PPIs for the rest of their life. An operation to strengthen the muscle at the bottom of the oesophagus, called a fundoplication, can also be performed, often using keyhole surgery techniques. Other treatments include removing the affected area (called endoscopic mucosal resection) using an endoscope, or alternatively a surgical resection, where a more extensive area of the oesophagus is removed and rejoined to the stomach. Endoscopic radiofrequency ablation which uses heat to destroy abnormal cells is another option.[10]

- **Oesophageal cancer.** An estimated one to 5 per cent of people with Barrett's oesophagus develop oesophageal cancer[10A] (see Chapter 7, page 126). It can be removed and successfully treated if in the early stages. This is another reason why it's important not to ignore GORD symptoms and opt for close monitoring if you are diagnosed with Barrett's oesophagus.

Hiatus hernia

This is the medical name for when part of the stomach protrudes up into the chest through the opening (a hiatus) in the diaphragm, a large sheet of muscle between the chest and the abdomen. It's relevant to this chapter because it can cause GORD, with symptoms including a bitter taste in the mouth, heartburn and chest pain. Hiatus hernias are more common with age as muscles weaken (especially after the age of 50) and/or you are overweight or pregnant.

Treatment as described for GORD will help. If the hernia is large, surgical treatment done at laparoscopy to repair the hernia and form what is caused a fundoplication may relieve the symptoms.

Globus sensation

Put simply this feels like you've got a lump in your throat – even though you don't have one really. It's a sensation that can come and go and doesn't make eating or drinking difficult, but you may worry that it's caused by something sinister. It's surprisingly common, accounting for one in 20 referrals to ear, nose and throat (ENT) specialists.[11]

The most common cause is acid reflux from the stomach, which can lead to excessive throat clearing and a tickly cough, as well as the 'lump in the throat' sensation. Some people report their symptoms get worse and become more frequent when they are under stress.

Be reassured though that you don't have a physical lump in your throat. However, the doctor will want to be able to distinguish globus sensation from other more serious conditions. You may be referred for an endoscopy or an X-ray to be certain. Experts advise drinking plenty of liquids (between 1.5 and 2 litres of water a day), drinking water with meals and avoiding coffee, too much alcohol or tea and fizzy or acidic drinks. They also recommend avoiding throat clearing, learning how to relax and deal with stress and taking medication for acid reflux.[12]

Burping and belching

Some people joke that a burp is a mark of appreciation for a good meal – but actually, although it's entirely a natural, normal involuntary process – it can be embarrassing in social situations, particularly if it's a regular problem.

Burping is caused by swallowed air building up in the stomach – we all swallow air when we eat – but sometimes swallow too much. For instance sucking on hard sweets, chewing gum and carbonated fizzy drinks may all contribute to swallowing too much air. According to the American College of Gastroenterology[13] people who experience anxiety or who have badly fitting dentures which cause them to chew abnormally, and also those who suffer from post-nasal drip (where catarrh secretions from the nose and nasal sinuses drain into the pharynx (throat)) can also swallow too much air. People who suffer from GORD may also belch as they attempt to clear stomach acid that has backed up from their throat and then swallow more air triggering more belching. Another possible cause is gastritis (inflammation of the lining of the stomach).[14] The air is either belched out as a burp or passed into the colon where it eventually emerges from the rectum as flatulence (passing wind – see Chapter 9, page 13). Some people with IBS are reported to be more sensitive to gas and can suffer abdominal pains and cramps as a result of gas build-up.

To prevent excessive burping, the standard advice is to avoid swallowing too much air when eating – try eating and drinking slowly, avoid fizzy drinks, chewing gum and hard sweets, see your dentist if your dentures don't fit, and talk to your doctor about treatments for post-nasal drip, including antihistamines and decongestants, and medication for treating GORD and gastritis.

Peptic ulcers

As explained at the beginning of this chapter, a peptic ulcer is an umbrella term for both gastric (stomach) ulcers and duodenal ulcers (in the first part of the small intestine) and sometimes even in the oesophagus. It can be slightly confusing as some people just refer to all ulcers as stomach ulcers.

What are they and why are they included in a chapter on indigestion? Peptic ulcers are open sores that develop in the lining of the stomach. The stomach and oesophagus have a mucosal lining which is normally protected against damage from stomach acid and other chemicals. The stomach secretes bicarbonate at the surface of the mucosal lining to neutralise the acid secreted into the middle of the stomach.[15] But when the body's normal defence mechanisms aren't functioning properly, the acid damages the mucosal lining and an ulcer begins to form. These look like large mouth ulcers and can be 1 to 2 cm in diameter. They are a very common problems estimated to affect one in 10 people at some point in their lives.[16]

Contrary to popular belief, peptic ulcers are not caused by stress, drinking too much alcohol or a bad diet (although there is some evidence that these may make existing ulcers worse).The most common reasons for stomach acids to succeed in forming an ulcer are:

- bacterial infection called *Helicobacter pylori* (see page 124), which causes inflammation in the lining of the stomach and resets acid production to a higher level, and

- side effects from non-steroidal anti-inflammatory drugs (NSAIDs), including ibuprofen and aspirin, which interfere with gastric defences.

Other causes of ulcers include smoking and steroid drugs if taken with NSAIDs; Crohn's disease (see Chapter 6, page 104) and rare hormonal problems which result in too much acid being produced.

More about *H. pylori*

Helicobacter pylori's role in causing peptic ulcers was only discovered in 1982 (by the Australian doctors Barry Marshall and Robin Warren who were both later awarded the Nobel Prize in Medicine). This discovery has revolutionised treatment of peptic ulcers because they can now be treated and prevented with antibiotics.[17] Most people are unaware they have been colonised with *H. pylori* because it doesn't produce any symptoms and not everyone who is infected will develop peptic ulcers. *H. pylori* is thought to be picked up by most people as a baby and is so common that over half the world's population carry it as a so-called commensal (where bacteria benefit from living in the gut but humans are unaffected).

At the time of Marshall and Warren's discovery of *H. pylori*'s role in causing peptic ulcers, it was still commonly believed that stress and lifestyle factors were the major causes of ulcers and the medical community initially greeted their findings with scepticism and criticism, but it soon became clear that *H. pylori* causes 90 per cent of gastric ulcers and 80 per cent of duodenal ulcers.[18]

What are the symptoms of ulcers?

Ulcers can be tricky to identify and distinguish from other causes of indigestion or other more serious conditions such as stomach cancer, gallstones or inflammation of the stomach lining. One of the most common symptoms of a stomach ulcer is a burning/

griping pain in the centre of the abdomen – this can be felt from your neck down to your belly button and radiate through to your back, lasting a few minutes or much longer. (Some people describe it as a knife-like pain.) However, some people don't experience any pain and just have indigestion, heartburn or feel nauseous.[19] You may also find you experience loss of appetite and weight loss, or belch or bloat after eating fatty foods.

Symptoms can start several hours after eating and commonly wake people at night. Ulcers can cause daily symptoms and these will be relieved by antacids and acid-reducing drugs – but then so will GORD and simple acid indigestion.

Diagnosing and treating an ulcer

If you are experiencing persistent indigestion and/or pain which is having an impact on your quality of life, see your doctor about your symptoms. It may well be simple indigestion but by taking a history and asking you questions, your doctor will be able to decide if your symptoms warrant further investigation.

Your doctor may decide it is simpler to test you for *H. pylori* and prescribe antibiotics to kill the bacteria if the test is positive, rather than order an endoscopy (see Glossary, page 181). However, an endoscopy is the procedure that is most certain to show if an ulcer is present. Other *H. pylori* tests include a special breath test, which can reveal high levels of carbon dioxide in *H. pylori* infection, and stool tests to detect the bacterial protein. Blood tests are also sometimes used but these will remain positive after eradication of the bacteria so the stool test (which detects current infection) has mostly replaced this.

The ulcers should heal within a few weeks with the usual triple therapy, which comprises treatment with two antibiotics, usually for a week, and a PPI for a while longer. This treatment with antibiotics is effective in 90 per cent of cases (remember to finish the course) and ulcers do not usually recur because the *H. pylori* bacterium has been eradicated. In the short term, the antibiotics possibly can cause bloating and diarrhoea and if you know you are allergic to penicillin, you must let your doctor know so you can be given an alternative.

If your doctor suspects your ulcer has been caused by NSAIDs you will usually be treated with PPIs to reduce acid secretion and alternative pain killers may be suggested, such as paracetamol. However, if your NSAIDs or aspirin can't be stopped you may be prescribed a PPI long term to avoid an ulcer recurring.

Giving up smoking can also reduce your chance of ulcers recurring.

If your symptoms come back after the course of triple therapy to eradicate the *H. pylori*, it may be that another condition such as GORD has been helped for a while by the course of PPIs, or it may be that you are one of the small percentage of people not successfully cleared on the first attempt. A further stool test (you need to wait six weeks to be certain) may show that the *H. pylori* is back. Alternative courses of antibiotics can then be tried until eradication is successful (see page 140-1 for NICE guidelines on cancer referral for stomach cancer).

Complications of ulcers

Some ulcers become more problematic and cause more serious complications. These complications include bleeding, a leak of contents through a perforating ulcer, and gastric obstruction blocking the passage of food due to the ulcer swelling and the formation of scar tissue.

Bleeding happens when an ulcer develops at the site of a blood vessel and is the most common complication, affecting around 15 per cent of people who develop ulcers.[20, 21] Symptoms of bleeding can include anaemia symptoms – breathlessness, fatigue and heart palpitations – or those caused by more sudden blood loss, including vomiting blood (called haematemesis) or passing stools which are black and tar-like (called melaena). These latter symptoms are a medical emergency so you need to seek urgent medical attention at an A&E/ emergency room or call for an ambulance. You will most likely be given an endoscopy to find the cause of your bleeding and treatment to stop the bleeding and/or a blood transfusion, although there are sometimes good reasons that can help avoid doing this unnecessarily.

If your ulcer perforates through the stomach or duodenum, it can cause sudden abdominal pain that gets rapidly worse and needs urgent admission to hospital. Perforation causes bacteria that normally inhabit the stomach to infect the lining of the abdomen – known as peritonitis. This is very serious because the bacteria can then spread into the bloodstream (sepsis) and spread to other organs, carrying the risk of multiple organ failure and death if untreated. Surgery may be needed.

Symptoms of gastric outlet obstruction due to ulcers include: repeated bouts of vomiting, persistent bloating and feeling full, and unexplained weight loss. Treatment options include a course of PPIs or H2-receptor antagonists to reduce inflammation. Other treatments include surgery to remove scar tissue causing obstruction and passing an endoscope down into the stomach or inflating a balloon to widen the site of the obstruction.

Gallstones

Gallstones are solid lumps that form in bile. Bile is made in the liver to digest fat and is stored in the gall bladder before secretion into the duodenum. Gallstones start as tiny crystals, growing into small and then larger stones. Most contain cholesterol, a waxy substance made in the liver.[21A]

Gallstones are an increasingly common problem in Western societies, including Europe and the US, where prevalence is estimated to be 10 to 15 per cent.[22] Various studies have shown more cases of gallstones are now being reported – and it is now the leading cause of hospital admission relating to gastro-intestinal symptoms in the US.[23]

The rise may be related in changes to diet in the West in the past two generations (higher calorie intake and fat content) and rising obesity levels. This is part of the increasingly common metabolic problems being encountered, leading a recent paper[24] to comment, 'The rising epidemic of obesity and metabolic syndrome predicts an escalation of cholesterol gallstone frequency.'

In the West most gallstones are formed predominantly from cholesterol. The rest are black pigment stones, formed from calcium bilirubinate, often due to an underlying medical condition with production of too much bilirubin, a waste product that comes from broken down red blood cells. This can make the skin and whites of the eyes appear yellow.

What are the symptoms?

Experts estimate that two out of three people who have gallstones don't have any symptoms (so-called 'silent' gallstones).

Gallstones usually only cause problems if they move from the gall bladder into the bile ducts (tubes that lead from the gall bladder and intestine). If they become lodged in the duct this can cause pain – known as biliary colic – which can be excruciating. The pain is felt in the top of the stomach, centrally or just under the ribs to the right-hand side. It usually feels much more uncomfortable than indigestion – people describe it as a griping pain which can come in waves and is severe enough for most people to seek medical help. The pains can last for a few hours and then usually go away. Sometimes this pain is confused with that of a myocardial infarction (a 'heart attack') so an ECG and other tests may be needed to rule this out.

If the stones block the main bile duct from the liver into the intestine, they can not only cause pain but also block bile flow and lead to jaundice, which means the body is unable to get rid of the bilirubin (see above). Sometimes gallstones are associated with acute pancreatitis, where the pancreas becomes inflamed, and patients experience severe upper abdominal pain, sometimes left sided or going into the back, and usually with nausea and vomiting. Acute pancreatitis will be diagnosed initially with a simple blood test (serum amylase).

Who gets them?

Gallstones tend to be more common in women; this is thought to be because the female sex hormone oestrogen increases cholesterol secretion and diminishes bile acid secretion. Women are almost twice as likely to develop gallstones as men, although the gap closes after the menopause.[25] Using the contraceptive pill and oestrogen hormone replacement therapy (HRT) are also regarded as risk factors for gallstones, as is pregnancy. According to the digestive disease charity Core, there's also some truth in the old saying that gallstones affect people with all the Fs – that's fair, female, forty and fertile – as they tend to be more common in women who are overweight and who have had children. Nowadays, though, gallstones are being diagnosed in much younger people, sometimes even in their teens,[21A,26] although as a general rule they are more common in older people.

Ethnic group and genetics are also important risk factors for gallstones. Prevalence of gallstones is highest amongst American Indian women (62–73 per cent), Canadian Indians (62 per cent) and lowest in Eastern countries such as Thailand (4 per cent), Japan (5 per cent) and China (15 per cent).[27] Studies have revealed that there is a five times elevated risk of developing gallstones in relatives of patients with gallstones.[28] These rates are higher in twins, with a 12 per cent increased risk in identical twins and 6 per cent increased risk in non-identical twins.[29] Several genes have been identified associated with stone formation, but experts say it's a complex interaction of genes *and* environmental factors.

Another risk factor for gallstones is getting older, with cases increasing dramatically over the age of 40. Type 1 diabetes and the metabolic syndrome (defined as having at least three features out of abdominal obesity, high blood pressure, high fasting blood glucose, increased triglyceride levels and reduced HDL cholesterol levels) also carry an increased risk of developing gallstones.[30]

Obesity is another important risk factor for gallstones. Studies have shown that at least one in four morbidly obese people have gallstones.[31] If you are obese in your late teens than you are particularly at risk.

Rapid weight loss from low-calorie diets or from bariatric (obesity) surgery are both associated with gallstones. Various studies estimate that 30 to 71 per cent of people in these groups will develop gallstones.[32, 33] However, only 7 to 16 per cent of people who develop gallstones after rapid weight loss will develop symptoms – this is best predicted by a weight loss of 25 per cent of body weight or more.[34]

When it comes to which foods influence gallstone formation, the evidence is less clear cut. Diets high in cholesterol, fatty acids, carbohydrates or legumes seem to increase the risk of cholelithiasis (formation of gallstones).[35, 36, 37] Unsaturated fats, coffee, vitamin C, calcium and moderate alcohol consumption seem to reduce the risk. Experts believe it's the shift to the Western-style diet with its high refined carbohydrate and fat content and low fibre element which offers the best explanation for the increase in cholesterol gallstones; these views came from studies amongst the American Indian population and in European countries following World War II.[38]

Other associations with gallstones include underlying chronic diseases such as liver diseases, Crohn's diseases, cystic fibrosis and sickle cell disease (pigment stones), as well as the side effects of some drugs including some thiazide diuretics and an antibiotic called ceftriaxone.

How are they diagnosed?

Gallstones usually show up very clearly on simple ultrasound scans of your abdomen. They may be picked up on CT or MRI scans. Your doctors may also run blood tests looking for inflammation or jaundice.

Treatment

If your gallstones aren't causing any symptoms you may not need any treatment at all. Even if you've had one attack it doesn't necessarily mean you'll have another in the near future or ever at all. The stone that blocked a duct may have been passed naturally out of the body without the need to remove it surgically or via an endoscope.

When stones are causing ongoing problems though, and need to be removed, doctors recommend removal of the gall bladder. You can manage without one with no problems – bile will just flow into the intestine. Some animals do not have a gallbladder at all.

The most commonly used method for removing the gallbladder involves keyhole surgery – a procedure called laparoscopic cholecystectomy (see Glossary, page 180).

If stones have entered the bile ducts, removal of the stones using an endoscope will be necessary. This procedure is called endoscopic retrograde cholangiopancreatography (ERCP) – see Glossary, page 182.

Chapter 9

Trouble down below

- Constipation
- Laxatives
- Piles (haemorrhoids) anal fissures
- Diverticulitis/diverticular disease
- The Bristol stool test

Constipation

What's normal and what's not?

Lots of people worry about their bowel movements and whether they are emptying their bowel regularly or not; it's a source of anxiety, particularly among older people, as constipation becomes more common as you get older due to ageing and the increased likelihood of being on medication which has 'constipating' side effects.

The truth is there's no real consensus on exactly how many bowel movements you should have in a day or a week – most people will have one or two a day – but some people will have more and others fewer. It's about what's normal for you.

If you want to get technical, according to the Rome criteria[1] constipation is defined as having a bowel movement less than three times a week. Medics define constipation as 'defecation which is unsatisfactory' based on infrequent stools, difficult stool passage, feeling that you haven't emptied your bowels and stools which are dry and hard and may be abnormally large or small.[2]

One thing's for sure though, getting constipated is a common complaint. It's hard to give accurate figures as definitions of constipation still vary worldwide, but one study[3] says rates vary between 2 and 27 per cent of the population. Another study of American adults put the figure at between 3 and 30 per cent of the population, with an average of 15 per cent.[4] In one study 45 per cent of participants had constipation symptoms that continued for five years.[5]

Other experts estimate constipation affects one in seven adults and one in three children.[6] Constipation is also very common in childhood; the continence charity ERIC (Education and Resources for Improving Childhood Continence) says constipation affects 29 per cent of under four-and-a-half-year-olds and 27.5 per cent of under nine-year-olds.

Every year a significant number of people get sufficiently uncomfortable and worried about constipation to see a doctor. This is reflected in prescriptions for laxatives – with 18.5 million prescriptions being made out for people in England in 2010.[7] On top of this, another £58 million is spent on 15.8 million over-the-counter laxative products from chemists for constipation.[8]

Who gets constipated?

Whilst constipation affects both sexes and all age groups (including babies and children) there are particular groups of people who seem to suffer from it more. For example, women are twice as likely to suffer from constipation as men.[9] It's also more common in older people; one study puts the figure at 26 per cent for women over 65 and 16 per cent for men over 65.[10] The figure rises to 34 per cent for women over 85 and 26 per cent for men in the same age group. As many as 80 per cent of people living in care homes may suffer from constipation.[11]

But it's not just the elderly who can get constipated – it really does affect all age groups. Pregnant women are also commonly affected by constipation with around 40 per cent complaining of problems with bowel movements.[12]

Are there different types of constipation?

There are two main types of constipation – the first is functional constipation without a known cause and the second is secondary constipation caused by either drug side effects or an underlying medical condition. Functional constipation is often diagnosed by eliminating secondary causes.

Secondary causes of constipation

There are a number of drugs which can cause constipation as a side effect, so your doctor may be able to change your medication if this is the case or give you lifestyle/dietary advice to try and counter its effects.

With increasing poly-pharmacy, where many patients over 65 are now on a cocktail of daily pills for long-term chronic conditions, and for preventing other health conditions such as heart disease, it is possible to be taking a number of drugs which have constipating effects so the effects are magnified (see Box 9.1).

Box 9.1 Drugs with constipating effects

The most common drugs (in no particular order) with constipating effects are:

- Aluminium antacids
- Antimuscarinics (such as procyclidine, oxybutynin)
- Antidepressants (most commonly tricyclic antidepressants, but others may cause constipation in some individuals)
- Some antiepileptics (for example, carbamazepine, gabapentin, oxcarbazepine, pregabalin, phenytoin)
- Sedating antihistamines (for hayfever and other allergies)
- Antipsychotics (used to treat anxiety)
- Antispasmodics (such as dicycloverine, hyoscine used to treat diarrhoea)
- Calcium supplements (often prescribed to women at risk of osteoporosis)
- Diuretics (water tablets prescribed to increase urine flow)
- Iron supplements (prescribed for anaemia)
- Opioids (opioid-based painkillers)
- Verapamil (for blood pressure complaints)

Source: NICE, 2015.[14]

Slow transit

In 15 to 30 per cent of cases of chronic constipation the cause is slow transit – put simply, the nerves and smooth muscle in the gut wall don't work efficiently and so don't propel food and waste at the normal speed. This can become apparent early in childhood or start later in life.

Experts say it can be a chicken-and-egg situation though, as in it's hard to know which comes first – the constipation causing slow transit or the slow transit causing constipation.

Slow transit is usually diagnosed by trying all the usual treatments such as more fluids, eating more fibre, laxatives and other drug treatments – and none of them working. Sometimes your doctor may order a transit study where you swallow small plastic markers and they are tracked by a series of X-rays to see how quickly they move through your gut to confirm the diagnosis.

In these cases eating more fibre overloads the bowel, which isn't working efficiently already and can't shift the fibre. Therefore, waste builds up in the colon causing constipation, bloating and pain. Many patients who eventually see a gastroenterologist about their constipation have been eating large amounts of fibre as instructed and it has done their symptoms no good and they complain it has actually made them worse.

Treatment options for slow transit include newer drugs called 5 HT4 receptor agonists (see below), and biofeedback – a combination of physical and psychological therapies designed to retrain the bowel and reintroduce regular bowel habits.

Medical conditions that can result in constipation

There are many medical conditions that can contribute towards constipation. These include endocrine (hormone) disorders such as type 1 diabetes; hypercalcaemia (too much calcium in the blood); hyperparathyroidism (a rare condition which causes hypercalcaemia); hypokalaemia (caused by low potassium levels); and hypothyroidism (a common condition of underactive thyroid). Other causes include neurological diseases such as multiple sclerosis, Parkinson's disease, spinal cord injuries and tumours.

Other causes of constipation can include structural abnormalities such as haemorrhoids and anal fissures (see page 168) and colonic strictures caused by diverticulitis (see page 175), inflammatory bowel disease (see Chapter 6), bowel cancer or cysts, rectal prolapse or prolapse after a third degree tear in childbirth. Another possibility is irritable bowel syndrome (see Chapter 3, page 25).

Usually you will have other symptoms suggestive of these underlying medical conditions and your doctor will have diagnosed your condition and be treating it.[15]

Treatments for constipation

If you see your doctor about short-term 'functional constipation' he or she is likely to give you appropriate diet and lifestyle advice to try and prevent it happening again and maybe laxatives in the short term to 'open you up' and get things moving again.

No investigations are routinely done unless constipation is believed to be secondary to another condition. So-called 'red flags' which will alert your doctor to other possible causes include blood in your stools (one symptom of colorectal cancer or a stomach ulcer, but more likely to be haemorrhoids); passing black tarry stools (possible causes include stomach ulcers or cancer) or light grey coloured stools (these can indicate a block in bile production and possible liver disease) and faecal incontinence. If you have one of these, you should be referred to a specialist.

If you are taking a drug which has a constipating effect this may be adjusted for you or an alternative drug prescribed.

Standard advice is to:

- **Increase the amount of dietary fibre in your diet.** Fibre is found in fruit, vegetables and grains. Aim to eat 18 to 30 g of fibre a day.[16] If your symptoms worsen, though, tell your GP, who may advise you to reduce your fibre intake if he/she suspects the cause of your constipation is slow transit (see page 162).

- **Ensure you have an adequate fluid intake.** The standard advice is eight to 10 glasses of water a day.

- **Get more physically active.** Being too sedentary can also contribute to constipation as it slows down metabolic processes including digestion.[17]

- **Eat fruits containing sorbitol.** Sorbitol is a natural sugar that is not absorbed well in the body and draws water into the gut. It's found in grapes, prunes, raisins, pears, plums, raspberries and strawberries and can be helpful in constipation.

Other self-help measures include getting into a regular routine – finding time to have bowel movements so you are not rushing and consequently ignoring the urge to pass a stool because you think you don't have time. Sometimes a better defaecation posture, raising your feet on a low block, can make things easier too.

However, sometimes diet and lifestyle measures don't have the desired effect or don't work quickly enough, so you may be prescribed an oral laxative to get things moving again.

The low down on laxatives

Laxatives are generally a short-term treatment to get the bowel moving again and can usually be stopped once stools are soft and regular again but some people may need them long term if they have a secondary cause for their constipation. Your doctor may mention to you that it can take several months to be successfully weaned off all laxatives. He or she will usually adjust the dose of laxatives gradually upwards (or downwards) to produce one or two soft, formed stools per day.

There are several different types of laxative – some can be bought over the counter and others are prescription-only from your GP.

- **Bulk-forming laxatives.** These are usually recommended in the first instance (except where constipation is due to opioid painkillers in the elderly in which case a combination of osmotic and stimulant laxatives may be prescribed – see below). Bulk-forming laxatives include ispaghula husk (psyllium), methylcellulose and sterculia and they work by helping your stools absorb fluid so they are less likely to dry out and become hard and difficult to pass. They are a good option if eating enough fibre is difficult for whatever reason and will provide a known, definite amount of fibre every day irrespective of what you eat. You need to make sure that you drink enough fluids with bulk-forming laxatives to avoid intestinal obstruction. They are best taken with meals to mix with the stool and can take two to three days to have an effect.[18]

- **Osmotic laxatives.** These are usually given to people who still have hard stools even after taking bulk-forming laxatives and following dietary and lifestyle advice. Osmotic laxatives retain water in the stool and make it softer and easier to pass. Lactulose is a non-absorbed sugar; it is sweet tasting but can cause bloating and colic. Magnesium salts such as Milk of Magnesia (magnesium hydroxide) have been used for a long time. Although large purgative doses are not advised, regular daily amounts (perhaps a 5 ml teaspoonful with your main meal) seem to work well and are safe and cheap. Mineral waters containing magnesium have also been shown to help. The synthetic polymers known as macrogols are regarded by some as the first choice prescribed osmotic laxative to try and are safe but more expensive.[19] They take two to three days to work and are beneficial at clearing the bowel initially.

- **Stimulant laxatives.** This type of laxative works as the name suggests by stimulating the muscles that line your digestive tract to move stools and waste products. They include senna, bisacodyl and sodium picosulphate. Senna takes eight to 12 hours to work, bisacodyl and sodium picosulphate six to 12 hours. These are commonly used, sometimes as over-the-counter natural products. Unfortunately, the body gets used to them and bigger doses will be needed over time.

- **Rectal laxatives (suppositories).** These are laxatives which are placed into the rectum and work very quickly within 15–30 minutes. These are usually reserved for cases of faecal impaction where the stools have hardened and are stuck in the rectum or where other laxatives have failed to have enough of an effect. Because they act so quickly though, some people find using them quite unpleasant and undignified.[20] Rectal laxatives include glycerol suppositories, sodium phosphate and docusate sodium enema.

- **5 HT4 receptor agonist.** A relatively new drug called prucalopride (Resolar) is sometimes used in the treatment of chronic constipation in adults for whom other laxatives haven't worked. It works by stimulating cells containing serotonin receptors in the intestine. They are involved in moving the contents of the intestines through the colon (the process known as peristalsis, see Chapter 1) so the bowel can be emptied. The drug mimics the effects of serotonin acting on the receptors and increasing muscular contractions of the intestine. However, the drug causes side effects in one in 10 people, including diarrhoea, nausea, headache and abdominal pain, and should be used with caution in frail people with specific medical conditions and, in some people with certain conditions, cannot be used at all.

• **Lubisprostone**. This is another new type of laxative for chronic idiopathic (no obvious cause) constipation which acts locally to increase intestinal fluid secretion. It can only be prescribed for you if you have tried at least two types of prescription laxatives at the highest dose for six months.[21]

Haemorrhoids (piles)

Haemorrhoids, or piles, are swollen blood vessels inside or outside the anus and rectum. The medical jargon for piles is 'enlarged swollen vascular mucosal cushions'. People say they can look like a bunch of grapes.

Although everybody has these haemorrhoidal veins, the exact cause of enlarged haemorrhoids is still not fully understood. They are thought to form as a result of constipation and straining, the effects of ageing and increased intra-abdominal pressure due to pregnancy.[22] Some people may also suffer a hereditary weakness in the venous walls.

Haemorrhoids inside the anus (internal haemorrhoids) are usually painless because there are no pain nerve fibres in this area; those that protrude outside can be itchy and painful and make your bottom feel sore and uncomfortable. It's possible to have both internal and external haemorrhoids at the same time.

Haemorrhoids are very common – estimates vary, but one study found they affected around 4.4 per cent of the US population and peak incidence was between the ages of 45 and 65.[23] Other studies of general practice records in England in the 1970s found they were more common with affluence.[24] The symptoms of piles often become noticeable after straining to pass a stool, during pregnancy and after giving birth, prolonged periods of sitting down (including travelling) and heavy lifting.

Symptoms

The symptoms of piles include rectal bleeding, usually when you pass a stool (you may notice bright red blood on toilet tissue when you wipe your bottom). The blood will be on the outside of the stool and not mixed in with it. Sometimes blood loss can be so extensive that people become anaemic. You may also experience anal itching and discharge of mucus. Other symptoms may include prolapse (where the piles hang down outside the anus) and pain (although, as we have said, internal haemorrhoids aren't usually painful unless the blood supply is cut off). Sometimes haemorrhoids can result in soiling.

Treating haemorrhoids

Thankfully, haemorrhoids aren't serious in most people and only 10 per cent of people ever need surgery. You can have haemorrhoids without symptoms so you may be unaware you have them.

Many people are able to manage their symptoms themselves by changing their diet and lifestyle habits to avoid constipation and straining (see page 165) and using haemorrhoid creams containing local anaesthetic they can buy over the counter from pharmacies for short-term pain relief.

However, if your symptoms persist it's best to see your doctor to check there isn't another more worrying cause for your rectal bleeding, such as bowel cancer or an underlying gut condition, such as inflammatory bowel diseases (see Chapter 6, page 105).

Is it piles or cancer?

Your doctor will take a history of your symptoms and then examine your back passage with a gloved finger to check for piles or any signs of other abnormalities.

Colorectal cancer

1.3.1 Refer adults using a suspected cancer pathway referral (for an appointment within 2 weeks) for colorectal cancer if:
- they are aged 40 and over with unexplained weight loss and abdominal pain or
- they are aged 50 and over with unexplained rectal bleeding or
- they are aged 60 and over with:
  o   iron deficiency anaemia or
  o   changes in their bowel habit, or
- tests show occult blood in their faeces (see recommendation 1.3.4 for who should be offered a test for occult blood in faeces). [new 2015]

1.3.2 Consider a suspected cancer pathway referral (for an appointment within 2 weeks) for colorectal cancer in adults with a rectal or abdominal mass. [new 2015]

1.3.3 Consider a suspected cancer pathway referral (for an appointment within 2 weeks) for colorectal cancer in adults aged under 50 with rectal bleeding and any of the following unexplained symptoms or findings:
- abdominal pain
- change in bowel habit
- weight loss
- iron deficiency anaemia. [new 2015]

1.3.4 Offer testing for occult blood in faeces to assess for colorectal cancer in adults without rectal bleeding who:
- are aged 50 and over with unexplained:
  - o abdominal pain or
  - o weight loss, or
- are aged under 60 with:
  - o changes in their bowel habit or
  - o iron deficiency anaemia, or
- are aged 60 and over and have anaemia even in the absence of iron deficiency. [new 2015]

If you have any 'red flag' symptoms you should be referred urgently to a specialist. The National Institute for Health and Care Excellence produced guidance on red flag symptoms – see opposite.

If your doctor identifies any of these red flag symptoms for possible cancer you will then undergo investigations in secondary care (see Chapter 7).

If your haemorrhoids are severe and already causing you a lot of pain and discomfort, you may also be referred on to a specialist. Also if your doctor suspects you may have symptoms of another medical condition such as diverticular disease, inflammatory bowel disease, polyps or Crohn's disease, he or she will refer you on to a gastroenterologist.

Conservative management of piles

In the majority of cases though, your doctor will give you advice about how to avoid constipation (see page 165) and straining and prescribe a haemorrhoid cream to provide short-term relief. If you are severely constipated he or she may also prescribe a laxative and suggest taking paracetamol for pain relief.

Other self-help measures include using moistened toilet tissue rather than dry toilet paper and taking care to gently pat the affected area dry.

Most people will never need specialist treatment for piles, but if you don't respond to these measures and your piles are having a significant impact on your quality of life you may need referral to a specialist (however trivial piles might seem to some).

Complications with piles

Sometimes piles are particularly nasty and can become ulcerated. Skin tags may also form and enlarge overlying skin causing hygiene problems and irritation. The skin around the anus may also become sore due to leaking mucus and fluid discharge. In rare cases, internal haemorrhoids can become engorged and this can lead to blood clots and severe pain. Other rare complications include perianal sepsis (sometimes leading to blood poisoning) and symptoms of anaemia resulting from persistent bleeding.

Seven ways to treat your haemorrhoid

Non-surgical treatments

- **Rubber band ligation (also called 'banding').** This involves applying an elastic band to the base of haemorrhoid to cut off the blood supply, causing it to wither away and eventually fall off (usually you won't notice this as it will happen during a bowel movement). Three can be treated at a time. The underlying tissue then heals. Complications can include haemorrhoid thrombosis, the band coming off with mild bleeding, and mucosal ulcers.

- **Injection sclerotherapy.** This procedure involves injecting phenol in oil in the lining of the rectum. It numbs the nerves, providing pain relief and also hardens the tissue so that scar tissue forms and within four to six weeks the haemorrhoids should shrivel up and disappear. Rare complications include pelvic infection.

- **Infra-red coagulation/photocoagulation.** Infra-red energy is used to burn the haemorrhoid tissue and cut off blood supply.

- **Bipolar diathermy and direct-current electrotherapy.** Electrical energy is used to apply heat to burn the haemorrhoid and cut off the blood supply.

Surgical treatments

As we've said above, only about one in 10 patients will need surgery for haemorrhoids. There are three commonly used procedures.

- **Haemorrhoidectomy.** This is an operation to cut out the haemorrhoids, usually under local anaesthetic. Its main drawback is that it is very painful after the operation and recovery can take a week. There's only a 5 per cent chance of the haemorrhoids growing back though. Complications can include passing blood clots, infection, urinary retention after the operation, and possibly faecal incontinence.

- **Stapled haemorrhoidopexy ('stapling').** This is used to treat prolapsed haemorrhoids. A stapling gun is used to staple the last section of the large intestine (the anorectum) and lift the haemorrhoids back into the canal. They are not cut out but just moved up the anal canal. Complications are rare but include sepsis, rectal perforation and haemorrhage.

- **Haemorrhoidal artery ligation.** A surgeon uses an internal Doppler ultrasound probe to locate the blood vessels in and around the anal canal and then each one is stitched closed to cut off the blood supply to the haemorrhoid. There is less pain after the operation and the hospital stay is shorter. NICE recommends the procedure as a 'safe and effective alternative' to haemorrhoidectomy and stapling.[26]

Anal fissures

Anal fissures are small tears or ulcers in the skin around your anus. They can cause a sharp, searing, burning pain when you have a bowel movement and for up to an hour afterwards. They may also bleed so you'll notice blood in the toilet or on your loo paper after you've passed a stool.

There are two main types:

- primary anal fissures with no obvious causes, and

- secondary anal fissures caused by constipation, with large hard stools causing a tear in the lining of the anal canal. Other possible causes include inflammatory bowel disease, pregnancy, bouts of diarrhoea and sexually transmitted disease.

They're common, affecting one in 10 people at some point during their lifetime and usually heal on their own without the need for specialist treatment. Your doctor will usually give you diet and lifestyle advice about avoiding constipation (see page 165) or suggest you use an anaesthetic cream, such as lidocaine.

Anal fissures can take a long time to go away as the pain causes reflex muscle spasm which reduces the blood supply needed to heal. To help this, you may be prescribed glyceryl trinitrate (GTN) cream to expand blood vessels in your anus to increase blood supply, speed up healing and relax the muscles inside the anus. Other treatments sometimes used include diltiazem cream, a calcium channel blocker medication, and botulium toxin injections, again to reduce the muscle spasm.

If the above approaches are ineffective you may need surgery. The most commonly performed operation for anal fissure is a lateral sphincterotomy where a small incision is made in the sphincter muscle (the ring of muscle surrounding the anal canal). It's a highly effective operation, but there is a 5 per cent risk with this procedure of losing some degree of bowel control and experiencing some faecal leakage.[27]

Diverticulosis, diverticular disease and diverticulitis

Diverticulosis becomes more common as you get older, affecting 25 per cent of people by the age of 60 and 66 per cent by the age of 85, making it one of the most common gastrointestinal conditions.[28] It's the medical name for the development of pouches extending from the wall of the large intestine, caused by weakness in the outer muscular layer. The inner layer of the intestine pushes through into the weaker outer muscular wall and forms a pouch called a diverticulum (plural diverticula). It can be diagnosed by colonoscopy or sigmoidoscopy, or picked up on CT scans or by other imaging techniques (see Glossary, page 181).

In most people diverticulosis doesn't have any symptoms, but in some people it leads to pain (often low down on the left-hand side), bloating and constipation/diarrhoea; this is referred to as diverticular disease.

If a diverticulum becomes inflamed this is known as diverticulitis and can lead to peritonitis. Symptoms of peritonititis include severe pain and tenderness in the lower abdomen, feeling sick and not passing urine for long periods. It may also be accompanied by a high temperature. Antibiotics can reduce the inflammation and sticking to fluids only until it settles, allowing your bowel to rest. Another complication is the formation of scar tissue which can cause blockages and bleeding – but these are rare. Sometimes bleeding can occur from diverticula but these complications of bleeding, perforation and stricturing are only problems in 1 per cent of the population.

If you have two or more attacks of diverticulitis then you might need surgery to remove the inflamed pouch and the rest of the section of the colon that is affected. The main reason why this surgery is done is to prevent further complications, such as an abscess forming either around the diverticula or elsewhere in the abdomen.

What causes diverticulosis?

It is widely believed that the Western-style low-fibre diet is the major cause of diverticulosis. The consensus after various studies in the 1960s – notably by Dr Denis Burkitt and also by Dr Neil Painter – argued that low fibre meant that the stool size and volume decreased and that diverticula formed as the intestines exerted more pressure to propel faeces through the gut. Not all studies, however, showed that dietary fibre intake is necessarily lower in people with asymptomatic diverticulosis.

Research studies have found that in patients who have symptoms of diverticulosis, a high-fibre diet *is* protective against diverticulitis.[29, 30] The EPIC study of British vegetarians found they had a 31 per cent reduced risk of diverticular disease compared with meat eaters. It found that both a vegetarian diet and a higher intake of fibre were significantly associated with a lower risk of diverticular disease and with reduced admission to hospital and death from diverticular disease.[31] These findings were reinforced by the Million Women Study in the UK,[32] which noted a reduction in diverticular disease in women on a high-fibre diet, although this found the risk was lowest in those who ate more fibre from fruit consumption rather than from grains.

There is now increasing interest in the genetic basis of diverticulosis – this is being investigated by assessing the health of migrants in their adopted countries to see if the environmental changes affect their gut health, as well as studies in twins. One study of Turkish migrants in a region of the Netherlands found there was no change in incidence of diverticular disease – which points towards genetic factors. Only 7.5 per cent of Turkish migrants were found to have diverticulosis compared with 50 per cent of native Dutch people.[33] A study of Swedish twins[34] estimated the heritability of diverticular disease was 40 per cent and the shared environmental causes accounted for 60 per cent. A Danish twin study put heritability of diverticular disease at 53 per cent. There are also a number of inherited diseases of connective tissue that are associated with diverticulosis, which have led researchers to believe diverticular disease and diverticulosis 'should be considered as a complex genetic disease resulting from environmental factors interacting with multiple susceptibility genes and disease modifiers'.[35] The authors say that, once identified, susceptibility genes may allow preventive screening and development of new drug treatments for diverticular disease.

These developments are still a long way off. At the moment, if you know you have diverticulosis in your family, it is probably best avoiding straining to pass your stools. Keep your stools soft with plenty of fruit and vegetables and think about the other laxatives we have discussed. Be sure to see your doctor if you develop new symptoms.

And finally...

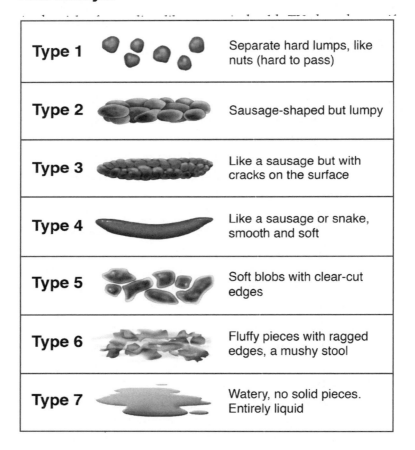

Type 1	Separate hard lumps, like nuts (hard to pass)
Type 2	Sausage-shaped but lumpy
Type 3	Like a sausage but with cracks on the surface
Type 4	Like a sausage or snake, smooth and soft
Type 5	Soft blobs with clear-cut edges
Type 6	Fluffy pieces with ragged edges, a mushy stool
Type 7	Watery, no solid pieces. Entirely liquid

Figure 9.1 The Bristol Stool Chart
© Rome Foundation (reproduced with permission)

Glossary

Abdomen: The abdomen is the part of the body below the chest and above the pelvis, and contains the kidneys and all the digestive organs, including the stomach, small and large intestines, pancreas, liver and gallbladder.

Acid reflux: Where acid from the stomach leaks up into the oesophagus (gullet).

Anus: Also referred to as the back passage. The opening at the end of the rectum where faeces are expelled from the body.

Barium enema: In this procedure, a fluid containing barium (a substance that is visible on X-rays) is inserted via a tube into your anus and large intestine. X-rays are then taken to show the lining of your bowel.

Barium swallow: The patient swallows a thick fluid containing barium (a substance that is visible on X-rays), which coats the lining of the oesophagus so it shows up on an X-ray.

Bile: Bile is a bitter, dark green or yellowish fluid made in the liver which helps break down fatty foods. It is stored in the gall bladder.

Biomarker: An abbreviation for 'biological marker'. Biomarkers indicate   the presence of a biological condition by measuring particular molecules.

Biopsy: The removal of small amounts of tissue from the body for further analysis.

Bowel: The bowel is made up of the small bowel (or small intestine, which is in turn made up of the duodenum, jejunum and ileum) and the large bowel (the colon and rectum). (See the diagram on page 12.)

Cholecystectomy: Removal of the gall bladder. The most common type of operation is **laparoscopic cholecystectomy**, which has a number of advantages over open surgery – the incision is smaller and there is less post-operative pain, a shorter hospital stay and quicker recovery. The old open-style cholecystectomy involved a six- to eight-inch incision and a hospital stay of five to seven days. These days it is usually reserved for patients who've had previous extensive abdominal surgery or who've had complications of gallstones such as gangrene or perforation of the gallbladder.

Colectomy: In this procedure, a section of the colon is removed and re-joined to another section of the normal bowel. It is rare to need a temporary or permanent colostomy (an external bag on the skin to collect the stool).

Colon: Also known as the large intestine, it is the next stage of the digestive system after the small intestine, beginning with the cecum, and continuing with the ascending colon, the transverse colon and the descending colon down to the sigmoid colon.

Colonoscopy: The patient is usually given a sedative and then a long narrow flexible telescopic camera is inserted into the anus and rectum to inspect the lining of the whole of the colon (also known as the large bowel/large intestine). The colon needs to be prepared with laxatives so the lining can be inspected fully. A **virtual colonoscopy** is a CT scan after special preparation to clear the colon. Once the colon is empty, gas is passed into your colon to enlarge it so small details can be seen.

CT scan: Computed tomography scan – a type of X-ray scan where multiple X-ray images taken from many angles are processed by computer to produce cross-sectional (tomographic) images of scanned areas.

CT urogram: A radioactive dye is injected into a vein and a CT scan is taken to give a detailed picture of the kidneys.

Duodenum: The first, small (roughly 12 inch) section of the small intestine/small bowel which occurs directly after the stomach, before the jejunum; here, the partly digested food (chyme) is mixed with secretions from the pancreas, liver and gallbladder. It can become inflamed, a condition known as **duodenitis**.

Dysentry: An infection of the large and small intestines which causes severe bloody diarrhoea, pain and fever.

Dyspepsia: Another name for indigestion.

Endocrine disorder: The endocrine system in the body makes hormones and when it goes wrong all sorts of conditions can result, including diabetes, thyroid disease, osteoporosis, stunted growth and infertility.

Endoscopy: A procedure where a microscopic camera on a

thin, flexible tube is inserted down through your mouth and the oesophagus, into your stomach and duodenum; or upward through your anus and rectum into your large bowel/intestine. You are usually given either a local anaesthetic or a sedative beforehand.

- An endoscopy through your mouth and throat is also known as an **upper gastrointestinal endoscopy**, or a **gastroscopy**, or a **oesophago-gastro-duodenoscopy.**

An alternative approach to an endoscopy is a **capsule endoscopy** which involves swallowing a capsule the size of a sweet. It contains a camera which takes pictures of the inside of the gut and transmits them to an external device. The capsule is then passed out of the body in a bowel movement.

Endoscopic retrograde cholangio-pancreatography (ERCP): An endoscope is passed down through the mouth into the stomach and into the duodenum. A tiny tube is passed down the endoscope into the bile duct and dye is squirted in for X-ray pictures. These can confirm if there is a gallstone or not. The stone will be removed or the bottom of the duct enlarged so the stone can pass out naturally. Avoiding the need for more extensive surgery is a big advantage, particularly if a patient is frail and/or elderly.

Epigastric mass: Lump or growth in the upper abdominal area.

Faecal calprotectin test: Stools are examined for levels of concentration of a protein called calprotectin, which is released in increased amounts when the bowel becomes inflamed, for example in ulcerative colitis or Crohn's disease.

Faeces: The solid waste matter remaining after digestion is completed.

Fine needle aspiration: A needle is used to drain fluid containing cells for analysis in a laboratory.

Flexible sigmoidoscopy: This procedure uses a shorter tube than a colonoscopy and just inspects the lower part of the large bowel (the sigmoid) and the rectum. This is a quick and safe procedure which needs little preparation.

FODMAPs: Stands for a group of short-chain carbohydrates called Fermentable Oligosaccharides, Disaccarharides and Monosaccharides, plus some sugar alcohols (Poloyols) that are found in various grains, vegetables, pulses and fruit. These have been implicated in irritable bowel syndrome and the recommendation is to try excluding them from the diet (see page 37).

Gall bladder: Stores bile, which is made in the liver and passes from it down the bile duct to the small intestine.

Gallstones: Cholelithiasis – the formation of solid lumps made from bile in the gall bladder.

Gastroenteritis: Inflammation of the stomach and large and small intestines, causing vomiting and diarrhoea.

Gastrointestinal digestive tract: The whole of the digestive tract from the stomach to the anus.

Gastroscopy: Another name for an upper endoscopy. The focus of attention is the stomach.

Glucose hydrogen breath test: Patients are given a drink containing glucose. Glucose should normally be absorbed quickly before any bacteria can break it down and form hydrogen – the body does not make hydrogen, only bacteria do. So if the amount of bacteria in the small intestine is high, the hydrogen content in your breath is increased and this can easily be detected by blowing into a machine.

Gullet: Another name for the oesophagus.

Gut: Another name for the gastrointestinal tract.

Gut biopsy: See endoscopy. A biopsy sample is taken at the same time as the endoscopy.

Gut microbiota: Also called gut microbiome: the millions of microbial organisms that exist throughout the gastrointestinal digestive tract.

Gut mucosa: The lining of the gastrointestinal digestive tract which absorbs the products of digestion and also plays an important role in the body's immune system, protecting from infection.

Heartburn: A burning sensation beneath the breastbone associated with, and often used as another name for, indigestion.

Ileal resection: This happens when an inflamed area of the ileum (the end part of the small intestine) is removed and the healthy tissue stitched back together.

Ileostomy: Waste is diverted from the ileum at the end of the small intestine to the exterior of the body via a stoma (an opening in the wall of the abdomen). In a **temporary ileostomy**, the small intestine is later re-attached to the colon. In a **permanent ileostomy** the colon is removed entirely and the stoma is either left in place, or an internal pouch is created to collect waste, which is then attached directly to the anus.

Ileum: The final section of the small intestine. This is where vitamin B12 is absorbed.

Indigestion: Also known as dyspepsia, acid reflux or heartburn, it is a burning sensation, heaviness or ache in the upper abdomen or lower part of the chest caused by an inflammation of the oesophagus.

Jejunum: The middle section of the small instestine.

Lactose hydrogen breath test: Patients are given a drink containing lactose, and then a breath test for hydrogen. If raised levels of hydrogen are detected it can be an indication that lactose is not being digested effectively or of abnormal bacteria in the gut.

Large intestine: Also called the colon or large bowel.

Microbiome: See Gut microbiota.

Mucosa: See Gut mucosa.

NSAIDs: Non-steroidal anti-inflammatory drugs, such as ibuprofen and aspirin.

Oesophagus: Also called the gullet, it is the long pipe that runs between your mouth and your stomach. It can become ulcerated by stomach acid, a condition called **oesophagitis**. If it is repeatedly ulcerated, the scar tissue can form **oesophageal strictures**, which can cause difficulty swallowing.

Pancreas: A gland organ that produces hormones and enzymes to break down food, and also insulin to regulate blood sugar. It can become inflamed, causing severe upper abdominal pain, a condition called **pancreatitis**.

Peristalsis: Wave-like muscle contractions which move food steadily through the oesophagus, the stomach and large and small intestines to the rectum.

Placebo effect: An effect which occurs when people believe they are having a treatment which will cure a condition and get better as a result, even though the treatment they received has no active ingredient that will affect their condition.

Pouch surgery: See ileostomy. This procedure is preferred to a **proctocolectomy with permanent ileostomy**, as patients can avoid permanent use of a bag. The colon and rectum are removed by the surgeon but the anus is left in place. The surgeon makes a pouch out of the lower end of the ileum and connects it to the anus. A temporary opening (stoma) is made in the abdominal wall to collect waste until the new pouch heals (usually within a few months).

PPIs: Proton pump inhibitors – drugs which reduce the production of stomach acid.

Prebiotics: A source of nourishment for probiotic bacteria in the intestines, comprising fibre compounds that are not destroyed in the digestive process.

Probiotics: Types of bacteria that aid the digestion of food in the large intestine.

Proctocolectomy with permanent ileostomy: This is the medical name for removal of the whole colon, rectum and anal canal. A permanent opening (a stoma) is made in the abdominal wall, usually on the lower right side on the abdomen, and the end of the lower small intestine (the ileum) brought through and joined to the skin. An external bag (sometimes referred to as an ileostomy bag) collects the waste from the stoma.

Rectum: The rectum is the chamber at the end of the large intestine where faeces are stored before being expelled through the anus.

Resection: This is where the surgeon removes inflamed sections of the gut and stitches the healthy tissue back together.

Resection with temporary ileostomy: Sometimes the gut just needs time to heal so waste is diverted away from it through a temporary stoma and the small intestine is re-attached to the colon at a later date.

SeHCAT test: This procedure involves swallowing a capsule containing selenium-labelled synthetic bile salt, which is safe as it contains about the same amount of radioactivity as we are all exposed to from natural background radiation sources every month, and then having two simple gamma camera scans, one on the day you swallow the capsule and another seven days later. It tests the function of the bowel by measuring how well the compound is retained or lost from the body.

Small bowel: See bowel. Also known as the small intestine.

Small intestine: See bowel. Also known as the small bowel.

Stomach: The first organ in the digestive process which takes food passed down through the mouth and oesophagus.

Stool: Another name for solid waste – see faeces.

Strictureplasty: The narrowed sections of the colon are opened up and reshaped/widened so that food is able to pass through easily.

Upper endoscopy: See endoscopy.

Villi: The fine 'fingers' which line the walls/mucosa of the gastrointestinal digestive tract, substantially increasing the effective digestive surface.

Virtual colonoscopy: See colonoscopy (page 181).

References

Chapter 1

1. Core (2015) Digesting the facts: what people are thinking about their digestive health. http://corecharity.org.uk/wp-content/uploads/2016/08/DigestingTheFactsReport.pdf (Accessed 3 August 2016)
2. The IBS Network. What is IBS? *The IBS Network*. 2016. https://www.theibsnetwork.org/ (accessed 31 May 2016).
2A. Soubiers A et al. Burden of IBS in an increasingly cost aware NHS. *Frontline Gastroenterology*. 24 February 2015. doi: 10.1136/flgastro-2014-100542.
3. Molodecky NA, Soon IS, Rabi DM, Ghali WA, Ferris M, Chernoff G, Benchimol EI, Panaccione R, Ghosh S, Barkema HW, Kaplan GG. Increasing incidence and prevalence of the inflammatory bowel diseases with time, based on systematic review. *Gastroenterology* 2012;142(1): 46-54. http://www.ncbi.nlm.nih.gov/pubmed/22001864 (accessed 19 February 2016).
4. BBC News. Rapid rise in Scots children with bowel diseases. *BBC News*. 13 June 2012. http://www.bbc.co.uk/news/uk-scotland-edinburgh-east-fife-18424572 (accessed 19 February 2016)
5. Coeliac UK. *Fourfold increase in the rate of diagnosed cases of coeliac disease in the UK*. Coeliac UK. 12 May 2014. https://www.coeliac.org.uk/document-library/1459-fourfold-increase-in-the-rate-of-diagnosed-cases-of-coeliac/ (accessed 31 May 2016).
6. Mintel. Gluten-free foods surge 63% in last two years. *Mintel*. 18

November 2014.
http://www.mintel.com/press-centre/food-and-drink/gluten-free-foods-surge-63-percent (accessed 22 February 2016).

7. Rostami K, Hogg-Kollars S. A patient's journey. Non-coeliac gluten sensitivity. *BMJ* 2012;30:345.
http://www.ncbi.nlm.nih.gov/pubmed/23204003 (accessed 22 February 2016).

8. Gibson PR, Shepherd SJ. Evidence-based dietary management of functional gastrointestinal symptoms: The FODMAP approach. *Journal Gastroenterology and Hepatology* 2010; 25(2):252-258.
http://onlinelibrary.wiley.com/doi/10.1111/j.1440-1746.2009.06149.x/pdf (accessed 22 February 2016).

10. AllergyUK. Dairy intolerance (including lactose intolerance). *AllergyUK*. October 2012
http://www.allergyuk.org/common-food-intolerances/dairy-intolerance#lactose-intolerance (accessed 22 February 2016).

11. Cancer Research UK. Bowel cancer statistics. *Cancer Research UK*. n.d.
http://www.cancerresearchuk.org/health-professional/cancer-statistics/statistics-by-cancer-type/bowel-cancer/incidence#heading-Two (accessed 31 May 2016).

12. Cancer Research UK. High risk groups for bowel cancer. *Cancer Research UK*. 20 January 2016.
http://www.cancerresearchuk.org/about-cancer/type/bowel-cancer/about/risks/high-risk-groups-for-bowel-cancer (accessed 22 February 2016).

13. Cancer Research UK. Stomach cancer symptoms. *Cancer Research UK*. 11 February 2014.
http://www.cancerresearchuk.org/about-cancer/type/stomach-cancer/about/stomach-cancer-symptoms (accessed 22 February 2016).

14. Cancer Research UK. Stomach cancer incidence trends over time. *Cancer Research UK*. 14 April 2016.
http://www.cancerresearchuk.org/health-professional/cancer-statistics/statistics-by-cancer-type/stomach-cancer/incidence#heading-Two (accessed 31 May 2016).

15. Bosshard W, Dreher R, Schnegg JF, Büla CJ. The treatment of chronic constipation in elderly people: an update. *Drugs Aging* 2004;21(14):911-30.
http://www.ncbi.nlm.nih.gov/pubmed/15554750 (accessed 22 February 2016).

16. Heitkemper MM, Chang L. Do fluctuations in ovarian hormones

affect gastrointestinal symptoms in women with irritable bowel syndrome? *Gend Med* 2009;6 (Suppl 2):152-67.
http://www.ncbi.nlm.nih.gov/pubmed/19406367 (accessed 22 February 2016).

17. Triadafilopoulos G, Finlayson M, Grellet C. Bowel dysfunction in postmenopausal women. *Women Health* 1998;27(4):55-66.
http://www.ncbi.nlm.nih.gov/pubmed/9796084 (accessed 22 February 2016).

18. Netdoctor. Constipation during pregnancy. *Netdoctor*. 25 February 2013.
http://www.netdoctor.co.uk/health_advice/facts/constipationpreg.htm (accessed 22 February 2016).

19. NHS Choices. Constipation – causes. *NHS Choices*. 24 December 2015.
http://www.nhs.uk/Conditions/Constipation/Pages/Causes.aspx (accessed 22 February 2016).

20. Patient. Acute Diarrhoea in adults. *Patient*. 1 December 2014.
http://www.patient.co.uk/doctor/acute-diarrhoea-in-adults-pro (accessed 22 February 2016).

21. Goodrich JK, Waters JL, Poole AC, Sutter JL, Koren O, Blekhman R, Beaumont M, Van Treuren W, Knight R, Bell JT, Spector TD, Clark AG, Ley RE. Human genetics shape the gut microbiome. *Cell* 2014; 159(4): 789-799.
http://www.sciencedirect.com/science/article/pii/S0092867414012410 (accessed 22 February 2016).

22. Picco MF. How long does it take to digest food — from the time you eat it to the time you excrete it? *Mayo Clinic*. 30 October 2012.
http://www.mayoclinic.org/digestive-system/expert-answers/faq-20058340 (accessed 22 February 2016).

23. NHS Choices. How's your gut? *NHS Choices*. 21 June 2014.
http://www.nhs.uk/livewell/digestive-health/pages/gut-health.aspx (accessed 22 February 2016)

Chapter 3

1.   Spiller R, Aziz Q, Creed F, Emmanuel A, Houghton L, Hungin P, Jones R, Kumar D, Rubin G, Trudgill N, Whorwell P. Guidelines on the irritable bowel syndrome: mechanisms and practical management. *Gut* 2007;56: 1770-1798. http://gut.bmj.com/content/56/12/1770 (accessed 22 February 2016).

2.   NICE. *Irritable bowel syndrome in adults: diagnosis and management.* NICE guidelines [CG61]. February 2008; updated February 2015. https://www.nice.org.uk/guidance/cg61 (accessed 22 February 2016).

3.   Hahn BA, Yan S, Strassels S. Impact of irritable bowel syndrome on quality of life and resource use in the United States and United Kingdom. *Digestion* 1999;60(1): 77-81. http://www.ncbi.nlm.nih.gov/pubmed/9892803 (accessed 22 February 2016).

4.   NHS Choices. Irritable bowel syndrome (IBS) – Symptoms. *NHS Choices.* 25 September 2014. http://www.nhs.uk/Conditions/Irritable-bowel-syndrome/Pages/Symptoms.aspx (accessed 22 February 2016).

5.   IBS Network. What is IBS. *IBS Network.* 2016. http://www.theibsnetwork.org/what-is-ibs/ (accessed 22 February 2016).

6.   BootsWebMD. Irritable bowel syndrome (IBS) symptoms. *BootsWebMD.* 23 May 2014. http://www.webmd.boots.com/ibs/guide/irritable-bowel-syndrome-ibs-symptoms (accessed 22 February 2016).

7.   NICE. *Irritable bowel syndrome in adults: diagnosis and management.* NICE guidelines [CG61]. February 2008; updated February 2015. http://www.nice.org.uk/guidance/cg61/chapter/1-recommendations (accessed 22 February 2016).

8.   NICE. *Irritable bowel syndrome in adults: diagnosis and management.* NICE guidelines [CG61]. February 2008; updated February 2015. http://www.nice.org.uk/guidance/cg61/chapter/1-recommendations (accessed 22 February 2016).

9.   Netdoctor. Irritable bowel syndrome (IBS). *Netdoctor.* 14 March 2014. http://www.netdoctor.co.uk/diseases/facts/irritablecolon.htm (accessed 22 February 2016).

10. Technische Universitaet Muenchen. Proof that a gut-wrenching complaint – irritable bowel syndrome – is not in your head.

ScienceDaily. 20 August 2010.
http://www.sciencedaily.com/releases/2010/08/100819141950.htm (accessed 22 February 2016).

11. The IBS Network. Is it all in my mind. *The IBS Network.* 2016.
http://www.theibsnetwork.org/the-self-care-plan/have-i-got-ibs/what-is-the-cause-of-my-ibs/is-it-all-in-my-mind/ (accessed 22 February 2016).

12. Marshall JK, Thabane M, Garg AX, Clark WF, Salvadori M, Collins SM. Incidence and epidemiology of irritable bowel syndrome after a large waterborne outbreak of bacterial dysentery. *Gastroenterology* 2006;131(2): 445-50.
http://www.ncbi.nlm.nih.gov/pubmed/16890598 (accessed 22 February 2016).

13. Neal KR, Barker L, Spiller RC. Prognosis in post-infective irritable bowel syndrome: a six year follow up study. *Gut* 2002;51: 410-413.
http://gut.bmj.com/content/51/3/410.full (accessed 22 February 2016).

14. Technische Universitaet Muenchen. Proof that a gut-wrenching complaint – irritable bowel syndrome – is not in your head. *ScienceDaily.* 20 August 2010.
http://www.sciencedaily.com/releases/2010/08/100819141950.htm (accessed 22 February 2016).

15. Whelan K. Probiotics and prebiotics in the management of irritable bowel syndrome: a review of recent clinical trials and systematic reviews. *Curr Opin Clin Nutr Metab Care* 2011;14(6): 581-7.
http://www.ncbi.nlm.nih.gov/pubmed/21892075 (accessed 22 February 2016).

16. Houghton LA, Lea R, Jackson N, Whorwell PJ. The menstrual cycle affects rectal sensitivity in patients with irritable bowel syndrome but not healthy volunteers. *Gut* 2002;50: 471-474.
http://gut.bmj.com/content/50/4/471.full (accessed 22 February 2016).

17. Triadafilopoulos G, Finlayson M, Grellet C. Bowel dysfunction in postmenopausal women. *Women Health* 1998;27(4): 55-66.
http://www.ncbi.nlm.nih.gov/pubmed/9796084 (accessed 22 February 2016).

17A. Shahbazkhani B et al. Non-celiac gluten sensitivity has narrowed the spectrum of irritable bowel syndrome: a double-blind randomized placebo-controlled trial. *Nutrients* 2015; 7(6):4542-4554. doi: 10.3390/nu7064542.

18. The IBS Network. Have I got a food allergy? *The IBS Network.* 2016.

http://www.theibsnetwork.org/the-self-care-plan/diet/have-i-got-a-food-allergy/ (accessed 22 February 2016).

19. Allergy UK/Alpro. *Dairy Intolerance: the trend towards self-diagnosis.* Allergy UK/Alpro. February 2013.
http://www.allergyuk.org/downloads/Corporate%20/Dairy-Intolerance-Report---Feb-2013-V3.pdf (accessed 22 February 2016).

20. BDA. Fact sheet: Irritable bowel syndrome and diet. *BDA.* January 2016.
https://www.bda.uk.com/foodfacts/IBSfoodfacts (accessed 22 February 2016).

21. Gibson PR, Shepherd SJ. Personal view: food for thought-western lifestyle and susceptibility to Crohn's disease. The FODMAP hypothesis. *Aliment Pharmacol Ther* 2005;21(12): 1399-409.
http://www.ncbi.nlm.nih.gov/pubmed/15948806 (accessed 22 February 2016).

22. Halmos EP, Power VA, Shepherd SJ, Gibson PR, Muir JG. A diet low in FODMAPs reduces symptoms of irritable bowel syndrome. *Gastroenterology* 2014;146(1): 67-75.
http://www.ncbi.nlm.nih.gov/pubmed/24076059. (accessed 22 February 2016).

23. Barrett JS, Gibson PR. Fermentable oligosaccharides, disaccharides, monosaccharides and polyols (FODMAPs) and nonallergic food intolerance: FODMAPs or food chemicals? *Therap Adv Gastroenterol* 2012; 5(4): 261-268.
http://www.ncbi.nlm.nih.gov/pmc/articles/PMC3388522/ (accessed 22 February 2016).

24. Hahn BA, Yan S, Strassels S. Impact of irritable bowel syndrome on quality of life and resource use in the United States and United Kingdom. *Digestion* 1999;60(1): 77-81.
http://www.ncbi.nlm.nih.gov/pubmed/9892803 (accessed 22 February 2016).

25. Whelan K. Probiotics and prebiotics in the management of irritable bowel syndrome: a review of recent clinical trials and systematic reviews. *Current Opinion in Clinical Nutrition & Metabolic Care* 2011;14(6): 581-587.
http://journals.lww.com/coclinicalnutrition/Abstract/2011/11000/Probiotics_and_prebiotics_in_the_management_of.11.aspx (accessed 19 April 2016).

26. Francis CY, Whorwell PJ. Bran and irritable bowel syndrome: time for reappraisal. *Lancet* 1994;344: 39–40.

27. Miller V, Lea R, Agrawal A, Whorwell PJ. Bran and irritable

bowel syndrome: the primary-care perspective. *Digestive and Liver Diseases* 2006;38: 737–740.

28. NICE. *Irritable bowel syndrome in adults: diagnosis and management Appendix A.* NICE guidelines [CG61]. February 2008; updated February 2015.
http://www.nice.org.uk/guidance/cg61/evidence/irritable-bowel-syndrome-guideline-addendum2 (accessed 22 February 2016).

29. Majid-Mahvi-Shirazi et al. IBS treatment: Cognitive behavioural therapy versus medical treatment. *Arch Med Sci* 2012; 8(1): 123–129.
http://www.ncbi.nlm.nih.gov/pmc/articles/PMC3309448/

30. Zernicke KA, Campbell TS, Blustein PK, Fung TS, Johnson JA, Bacon SL, Carlson LE. Mindfulness-based stress reduction for the treatment of irritable bowel syndrome symptoms: a randomized wait-list controlled trial. *Int J Behav Med* 2013 Sep;20(3): 385-96.
http://www.ncbi.nlm.nih.gov/pubmed/22618308 (accessed 22 February 2016).

31. NICE. *Irritable bowel syndrome in adults: diagnosis and management Appendix A.* NICE guidelines [CG61]. February 2008; updated February 2015.
http://www.nice.org.uk/guidance/cg61/evidence/irritable-bowel-syndrome-guideline-addendum2 (accessed 22 February 2016).

32. Simrén M, Barbara, G, Flint HJ, Spiegel BMR, Spiller RC, Vanner S, Verdu EF, Whorwell PJ, Zoetendal EG. Intestinal microbiota in functional bowel disorders: a Rome foundation report. *Gut* 2013; 62(1): 159–176.
http://www.ncbi.nlm.nih.gov/pmc/articles/PMC3551212/ (accessed 22 February 2016).

33. Saulnier DMA, Spinler JK, Gibson GR, Versalovic J. Mechanisms of probiosis and prebiosis: considerations for enhanced functional foods. *Curr Opin Biotechnol* 2009; 20(2): 135–141.
http://www.ncbi.nlm.nih.gov/pmc/articles/PMC2713183/ (accessed 22 February 2016).

34. Hoveyda N, Heneghan C, Mahtani KR, Perera R, Roberts N, Glasziou P. A systematic review and meta-analysis: probiotics in the treatment of irritable bowel syndrome. *BMC Gastroenterol* 2009; 9:15.
http://www.ncbi.nlm.nih.gov/pubmed/19220890 (accessed 20 May 2016).

35. Moayyedi P, Ford AC, Talley NJ, Cremonini F, Foxx-Orenstein AE, Brandt LJ, Quigley EM. The efficacy of probiotics in the treatment of irritable bowel syndrome: a systematic review. *Gut* 2010; 59:325–332.

http://www.ncbi.nlm.nih.gov/pubmed/19091823 (accessed 20 May 2016).

36. Whorwell PJ. Do probiotics improve symptoms in patients with irritable bowel syndrome? *Ther Adv Gastroenterol* 2009; 2(Suppl 1):S37–S44.

37. Brenner DM, Moeller MJ, Chey WD, Schoenfeld PS. The utility of probiotics in the treatment of irritable bowel syndrome: a systematic review. *Am J Gastroenterol* 2009; 104:1033–1049; quiz 1050. http://www.ncbi.nlm.nih.gov/pubmed/19277023 (accessed 20 May 2016).

38. McFarland LV, Dublin S. Meta-analysis of probiotics for the treatment of irritable bowel syndrome. *World J Gastroenterol* 2008; 14:2650–2661. http://www.ncbi.nlm.nih.gov/pubmed/18461650 (accessed 20 May 2016).

39. Brenner D, Moeller M et al. The utility of probiotics in the treatment of irritable bowel syndrome: a systematic review. *American Journal of Gastroenterology* 2009;104: 103–109.

40. Hungan APS, Mulligan C, Whorwell P, Agréus L, Fracasso P, Lionis C, Mendive J, Philippart de Foy J-M, Rubin G, Winchester C and Wit N. Systematic review: probiotics in the management of lower gastrointestinal symptoms in clinical practice – an evidence-based international guide. *Aliment Pharmacol Ther* 2013; 38(8): 864–886. http://www.ncbi.nlm.nih.gov/pmc/articles/PMC3925990/ (accessed 20 May 2016).

41. Didari T, Mozaffari S, Nikfar S, and Abdollahi M. Effectiveness of probiotics in irritable bowel syndrome: Updated systematic review with meta-analysis. *World J Gastroenterol* 2015; 21(10): 3072–3084. http://www.wjgnet.com/1007-9327/full/v21/i10/3072.htm (accessed 20 May 2016).

42. Floch MH, Walker WA, Madsen K, Sanders ME, Macfarlane GT, Flint HJ, Dieleman LA, Ringel Y, Guandalini S, Kelly CP and Brandt LJ. Recommendations for probiotic use-2011 update. *J Clin Gastroenterol* 2011;45 Suppl:S168-71. http://www.ncbi.nlm.nih.gov/pubmed/21992958/ (accessed 20 May 2016).

43. Guglielmetti S, Mora D, Gschwender M, Popp K. Randomised clinical trial: Bifidobacterium bifidum MIMBb75 significantly alleviates irritable bowel syndrome and improves quality of life-a

double-blind, placebo-controlled study. *Ailment Pharmacol Ther* 2011 May;33(10):1123-32.
http://www.ncbi.nlm.nih.gov/pubmed/21418261 (accessed 20 May 2016).

44. Shokryazdan P, Sieo CC, Kalavathy R, Liang JB, Alitheen NB, Jahromi MF and Ho YW. Probiotic potential of lactobacillus strains with antimicrobial activity against some human pathogenic strains. *Biomed Res Int* 2014; 2014: 927268.
http://www.ncbi.nlm.nih.gov/pmc/articles/PMC4106073/ (accessed 20 May 2016).

45. Zatorski H, Fichna J. What is the future of the gut microbiota-related treatment? Toward modulation of microbiota in preventive and therapeutic medicine. *Front Med* 2014;1: 19.
http://www.ncbi.nlm.nih.gov/pmc/articles/PMC4335382/ (accessed 22 February 2016).

46. Whorwell PJ, Prior A, Faragher EB. Controlled trial of hypnotherapy in the treatment of severe refractory irritable-bowel syndrome. *Lancet* 1984;2(8414): 1232-4.
http://www.ncbi.nlm.nih.gov/pubmed/6150275 (accessed 22 February 2016).

47. Lindfors P, Unge P, Arvidsson P, Nyhlin H, Björnsson E, Abrahamsson H, Simrén M. Effects of gut-directed hypnotherapy on IBS in different clinical settings-results from two randomized, controlled trials. *American Journal of Gastroenterologists* 2012; 107 (2); 276-285.
http://www.ncbi.nlm.nih.gov/pubmed/?term=American+Journal+of+Gastroenterologists+2012%3B+107+%282%29%3B+276-285. (accessed 24 May 2016).

48. Lee HH, Choi YY, Choi M-G. The Efficacy of Hypnotherapy in the Treatment of Irritable Bowel Syndrome: A Systematic Review and Meta-analysis. *J Neurogastroenterol Motil* 2014; 20(2): 152–162.
http://www.ncbi.nlm.nih.gov/pmc/articles/PMC4015203/ (accessed 19 April 2016).

49. Dong YY, Zuo XL, Li CQ, Yu YB, Zhao QJ, Li YQ. Prevalence of irritable bowel syndrome in Chinese college and university students assessed using Rome III criteria. *World J Gastroenterol* 2010;16(33): 4221-6.
http://www.ncbi.nlm.nih.gov/pubmed/20806442/ (accessed 22 February 2016).

50. Pedersen N, Andersen NN, Végh Z, Jensen L, Ankersen DV, Felding M, Simonsen MH, Burisch J, Munkholm P. Ehealth: Low

FODMAP diet vs *Lactobacillus rhamnosus* GG in irritable bowel syndrome. *World J Gastroenterol* 2014;20(43): 16215–16226. http://www.ncbi.nlm.nih.gov/pmc/articles/PMC4239510/ (accessed 22 February 2016).

51. Peckham EJ, Nelson EA, Greenhalgh J, Cooper K, Roberts ER, Agrawal A. Homeopathy for treatment of irritable bowel syndrome. *Cochrane Database Syst Rev* 2013;11: CD009710. http://www.ncbi.nlm.nih.gov/pubmed/24222383 (accessed 22 February 2016).

52. Drinkaware. Is alcohol harming your stomach? *Drinkaware.* April 2015. https://www.drinkaware.co.uk/check-the-facts/health-effects-of-alcohol/effects-on-the-body/is-alcohol-harming-your-stomach (accessed 22 February 2016).

Chapter 4

1. Mintel. Gluten-free foods surge 63% in last two years. *Mintel.* 18 November 2014.
    http://www.mintel.com/press-centre/food-and-drink/gluten-free-foods-surge-63-percent (accessed 19 April 2016).

2. Rona RJ, Keil T, Summers C, Gislason D, Zuidmeer L, Sodergren E, Sigurdardottir ST, Lindner T, Goldhahn K, Dahlstrom J, McBride D, Madsen C. The prevalence of food allergy: a meta-analysis. *J Allergy Clin Immunol* 2007;120(3): 638-46.
    http://www.ncbi.nlm.nih.gov/pubmed/17628647 (accessed 23 February 2016).

3. Shiner M. Coeliac disease: histopathological findings in the small intestinal mucosa studied by a peroral biopsy technique. *Gut* 1960;1: 48-54.
    http://gut.bmj.com/content/1/1/48.full.pdf (accessed 23 February 2016).

4. Genetics Home Reference. Celiac disease. *Genetics Home Reference.* September 2015.
    http://ghr.nlm.nih.gov/condition/celiac-disease (accessed 23 February 2016).

5. World Gastroenterology Organisation. *Global Guidelines: Celiac disease.* World Gastroenterology Organisation. April 2012.
    http://www.worldgastroenterology.org/assets/export/userfiles/2012_Celiac%20Disease_long_FINAL.pdf (accessed 23 February 2016).

6. World Gastroenterology Organisation. *Global Guidelines: Celiac disease.* World Gastroenterology Organisation. April 2012.
    http://www.worldgastroenterology.org/assets/export/userfiles/2012_Celiac%20Disease_long_FINAL.pdf (accessed 23 February 2016).

7. Core. Information about Coeliac disease. *Core.* 2014.
    http://beta.corecharity.org.uk/wp-content/uploads/2015/10/Core-Patient-Information-Coeliac-Disease.pdf (accessed 23 February 2016).

8. Coeliac UK. Coeliac disease key facts and stats. *Coeliac UK.* 14 May 2013.
    https://www.coeliac.org.uk/document-library/25-key-facts-and-stats/ (accessed 19 April 2016).

9. Coeliac UK. Dermatitis herpetiformis. *Coeliac UK.* 26 June 2013.
    https://www.coeliac.org.uk/coeliac-disease/about-coeliac-disease-and-dermatitis-herpetiformis/dermatitis-herpetiformis/ (accessed 23 February 2016).

10. World Gastroenterology Organisation. *Global Guidelines: Celiac disease*. World Gastroenterology Organisation. April 2012. http://www.worldgastroenterology.org/assets/export/userfiles/2012_Celiac%20Disease_long_FINAL.pdf (accessed 23 February 2016).

11. NICE. *Coeliac disease: recognition, assessment and management*. NICE guidelines [NG20]. 2 September 2015. https://www.nice.org.uk/guidance/ng20/resources/coeliac-disease-recognition-assessment-and-management-1837325178565 (accessed 1 August 2016).

12. West J, Fleming KM, Tata LJ, Card TR, Crooks CJ. Incidence and prevalence of celiac disease and dermatitis herpetiformis in the UK over two decades: population-based study. *Am J Gastroenterol* 2014; 109: 757–768. http://www.nature.com/ajg/journal/v109/n5/abs/ajg201455a.htmlttp://www.nature.com/ajg/journal/v109/n5/abs/ajg201455a.html (accessed 23 February 2016).

13. Gibert A, Espadaler M, Angel Canela M, Sánchez A, Vaqué C, Rafecas M. Consumption of gluten-free products: should the threshold value for trace amounts of gluten be at 20, 100 or 200 p.p.m.? *Eur J Gastroenterol Hepatol* 2006;18(11): 1187-95. http://www.ncbi.nlm.nih.gov/pubmed/17033440 (accessed 23 February 2016).

14. World Gastroenterology Organisation. *Global Guidelines: Celiac disease*. World Gastroenterology Organisation. April 2012. http://www.worldgastroenterology.org/assets/export/userfiles/2012_Celiac%20Disease_long_FINAL.pdf (accessed 23 February 2016).

15. Murch S, Jenkins H, Auth M, Bremner R, Butt A, France S, Furman M, Gillett P, Kiparissi F, Lawson M, McLain B, Morris M-A, Sleet S, Thorpe M. Joint BSPGHAN and Coeliac UK guidelines for the diagnosis and management of coeliac disease in children. *Arch Dis Child* 2013;98: 806-811. https://bspghan.org.uk/documents/Static/Coeliac%20Guidelines%202013.pdf (accessed 23 February 2016).

16. NICE. *Coeliac disease: recognition and assessment*. NICE guidelines [CG86]. May 2009. http://publications.nice.org.uk/coeliac-disease-recognition-and-assessment-of-coeliac-disease-ifp86/recognition-and-assessment (accessed 23 February 2016).

17. NICE. *Coeliac disease: recognition and assessment.* NICE guidelines [CG86]. May 2009. https://www.nice.org.uk/guidance/ng20/resources/coeliac-disease-recognition-assessment-and-management-1837325178565 (accessed 23 February 2016).

18. World Gastroenterology Organisation. *Global Guidelines: Celiac disease.* World Gastroenterology Organisation. April 2012. http://www.worldgastroenterology.org/assets/export/userfiles/2012_Celiac%20Disease_long_FINAL.pdf (accessed 23 February 2016).

19. Coeliac UK. Gut biopsy. *Coeliac UK.* nd. https://www.coeliac.org.uk/coeliac-disease/getting-diagnosed/gut-biopsy/ (accessed 23 February 2016).

20. World Gastroenterology Organisation. *Global Guidelines: Celiac disease.* World Gastroenterology Organisation. April 2012. http://www.worldgastroenterology.org/assets/export/userfiles/2012_Celiac%20Disease_long_FINAL.pdf (accessed 23 February 2016).

21. World Gastroenterology Organisation. *Global Guidelines: Celiac disease.* World Gastroenterology Organisation. April 2012. http://www.worldgastroenterology.org/assets/export/userfiles/2012_Celiac%20Disease_long_FINAL.pdf (accessed 23 February 2016).

22. Elli L, Roncoroni L, Bardella MT. Non-celiac gluten sensitivity: Time for sifting the grain. *World J Gastroenterol* 2015; 21(27): 8221–8226. http://www.ncbi.nlm.nih.gov/pmc/articles/PMC4507091/ (accessed 23 February 2016).

23. Anonymous, Rostami K, Hogg-Kollars S. Non-coeliac gluten sensitivity. *BMJ* 2012;345. http://www.bmj.com/content/345/bmj.e7982 (accessed 23 February 2016).

24. Elli L, Roncoroni L, Bardella MT. Non-celiac gluten sensitivity: Time for sifting the grain. *World J Gastroenterol* 2015; 21(27): 8221–8226. http://www.ncbi.nlm.nih.gov/pmc/articles/PMC4507091/ (accessed 23 February 2016).

25. Sapone A, Bai JC, Ciacci C, Dolinsek J, Green PHR, Hadjivassiliou M, Kaukinen K, Rostami K, Sanders DS, Schumann M, Ullrich R, Villalta D, Volta U, Catassi C, Fasano A. Spectrum of gluten-related disorders: consensus on new nomenclature and classification. *BMC Med* 2012; 10: 13.

http://www.ncbi.nlm.nih.gov/pmc/articles/PMC3292448/ (accessed 23 February 2016).

26. Carroccio A, Mansueto P, Iacono G, Soresi M, D'Alcamo A, Cavataio F, Brusca I, Florena AM, Ambrosiano G, Seidita A, Pirrone G, Rini GB. Non-celiac wheat sensitivity diagnosed by double-blind placebo-controlled challenge: exploring a new clinical entity. *Am J Gastroenterol* 2012;107(12): 1898-906.
   http://www.ncbi.nlm.nih.gov/pubmed/22825366 (accessed 19 April 2016).

26A. Shahbazkhari B et al. Non celiac gluten sensitivity has narrowed the spectrums of irritable bowel syndrome. *Nutrients* 2015; 7(6): 4542-4554.

27. Biesiekierski JR, Newnham ED, Irving PM, Barrett JS, Haines M, Doecke JD, Shepherd SJ, Muir JG, Gibson PR. Gluten causes gastrointestinal symptoms in subjects without celiac disease: a double-blind randomized placebo-controlled trial. *Am J Gastroenterol* 2011;106(3): 508-14.
   http://www.ncbi.nlm.nih.gov/pubmed/21224837 (accessed 23 February 2016).

28. Biesiekierski JR, Peters SL, Newnham ED, Rosella O, Muir JG, Gibson PR. No effects of gluten in patients with self-reported non-celiac gluten sensitivity after dietary reduction of fermentable, poorly absorbed, short-chain carbohydrates. *Gastroenterology* 2013;145(2): 320-8.
   http://www.ncbi.nlm.nih.gov/pubmed/23648697 (accessed 23 February 2016).

29. Biesiekierski JR, Iven J. Non-coeliac gluten sensitivity: piecing the puzzle together. *United European Gastroenterol J* 2015;3(2): 160–165.
   http://www.ncbi.nlm.nih.gov/pmc/articles/PMC4406911/ (accessed 23 February 2016).

29A. Catassi C, et al. Diagnosis of non-celiac gluten sensitivity: The Salerno Experts' Criteria. *Nutrients* 2015; 7(6): 4966-4977.

30. Catassi C et al. Diagnosis of non-celiac gluten sensitivity: the Salerno Experts' Criteria. *Nutrients* 2015; 7(6): 4966-4977.

31. NHS Choices. Should you cut out bread to stop bloating? *NHS Choices*. 18 May 2015.
   http://www.nhs.uk/livewell/digestive-health/pages/cutting-out-bread.aspx (accessed 23 February 2016).

Chapter 5

1. Pattni S, Walters JRF. Recent advances in the understanding of bile acid malabsorption. *Br Med Bull* 2009;Nov: 1-15. http://bmb.oxfordjournals.org/content/early/2009/11/08/bmb.ldp032.full (accessed 23 February 2016).

2. NICE. Potential benefits of a promising technology to diagnose bile acid malabsorption to be explored further in new research. *NICE*. 31 July 2012. https://www.nice.org.uk/news/press-and-media/potential-benefits-of-a-promising-technology-to-diagnose-bile-acid-malabsorption-to-be-explored-further-in-new-research (accessed 23 February 2016).

3. Wedlake L, A'Hern R, Russell D, Thomas K, Walters JR, Andreyev HJ. Systematic review: the prevalence of idiopathic bile acid malabsorption as diagnosed by SeHCAT scanning in patients with diarrhoea-predominant irritable bowel syndrome. *Aliment Pharmacol Ther* 2009;30(7): 707-17. http://www.ncbi.nlm.nih.gov/pubmed/?term=Systematic+review%3A+the+prevalence+of+idiopathic+bile+acid+malabsorption+%28+-BAM%29+as+diagnosed (accessed 23 February 2016).

4. NICE. Potential benefits of a promising technology to diagnose bile acid malabsorption to be explored further in new research. *NICE*. 31 July 2012. https://www.nice.org.uk/news/press-and-media/potential-benefits-of-a-promising-technology-to-diagnose-bile-acid-malabsorption-to-be-explored-further-in-new-research (accessed 23 February 2016).

5. Khalid U, Lalji A, Stafferton R, Andreyev J. Bile acid malabsoption: a forgotten diagnosis? *Clin Med (Lond)* 2010;10(2): 124-6. http://www.ncbi.nlm.nih.gov/pubmed/20437979/ (accessed 23 February 2016).

6. Fernández-Bañares F, Esteve M, Salas A, Alsina M, Farré C, González C, Buxeda M, Forné M, Rosinach M, Espinós JC, Maria Viver J. Systematic evaluation of the causes of chronic watery diarrhea with functional characteristics. *Am J Gastroenterol* 2007;102(11): 2520-8. http://www.ncbi.nlm.nih.gov/pubmed/17680846 (accessed 23 February 2016).

7. Slattery SA, Niaz O, Aziz Q, Ford AC, Farmer AD. Systematic review with meta-analysis: the prevalence of bile acid

malabsorption in the irritable bowel syndrome with diarrhoea. *Aliment Pharmacol Ther* 2015;42(1): 3-11.
http://ncbi.nlm.nih.gob/pubmed/25913530 (accessed 19 April 2016).

8. Islam RS, DiBaise JK. Bile acids: an underrecognized and underappreciated cause of chronic diarrhea. Nutrition Issues in Gastroenterology, Series #110. *Practical Gastroenterology* 2012; 32-44. https://med.virginia.edu/ginutrition/wp-content/uploads/sites/199/2014/06/Parrish_Oct_12.pdf (accessed 19 April 2016).

9. Pimentel M. A new IBS solution. *IBS Tales*. 23 February 2016. http://www.ibstales.com/a-new-ibs-solution.htm (accessed 23 February 2016).

10. Pimentel M. A new IBS solution. *Health Point Press*. N.d. http://www.anewibssolution.com/ (accessed 23 February 2016).

11. Pimentel M. Review of rifaximin as treatment for SIBO and IBS. *Expert Opin Investig Drugs* 2009;18(3): 349-58. http://www.ncbi.nlm.nih.gov/pubmed/19243285 (accessed 23 February 2016).

12. NIDDK. Microscopic colitis: collagenous colitis and lymphocytic colitis. *NIDDK* June 2014. http://www.niddk.nih.gov/health-information/health-topics/digestive-diseases/microscopic-colitis/Pages/facts.aspx (accessed 23 February 2016).

13. Kingham JG, Levison DA, Ball JA, Dawson AM. Microscopic colitis-a cause of chronic watery diarrhoea. *Br Med J (Clin Res Ed)* 1982;285(6355): 1601-4. http://www.ncbi.nlm.nih.gov/pubmed/6128051 (accessed 23 February 2016).

14. Tromm A. *Microscopic colitis: collagenous and lymphocytic colitis*. Falk Foundation eV. 2011. https://www.drfalk.co.uk/index.php/download_file/-/2902 (accessed 23 February 2016).

Chapter 6

1. Ng SC. Inflammatory bowel disease in Asia. *Gastroenterol Hepatol (N Y)* 2013;9(1): 28–30.
   http://www.ncbi.nlm.nih.gov/pmc/articles/PMC3975975/ (accessed 24 February 2016).

2. Bradford, E. NHS struggles with bowel disease 'epidemic'. *BBC News*. 17 May 2010.
   http://news.bbc.co.uk/1/hi/scotland/8684337.stm (accessed 24 February 2016).

3. Molodecky NA, Soon IS, Rabi DM, Ghali WA, Ferris M, Chernoff G, Benchimol EI, Panaccione R, Ghosh S, Barkema HW, Kaplan GG. Increasing incidence and prevalence of the inflammatory bowel diseases with time, based on systematic review. *Gastroenterology* 2012;142(1): 46-54.
   http://www.ncbi.nlm.nih.gov/pubmed/22001864 (accessed 24 February 2016).

4. Ahmad T, Tamboli CP, Jewell D, Colombel JF. Clinical relevance of advances in genetics and pharmacogenetics of IBD. *Gastroenterology* 2004;126(6): 1533-49.
   http://www.ncbi.nlm.nih.gov/pubmed/15168365/ (accessed 24 February 2016).

5. Molodecky NA, Kaplan GG. Environmental risk factors for inflammatory bowel disease. *Gastroenterol Hepatol (N Y)* 2010; 6(5): 339–346.
   http://www.ncbi.nlm.nih.gov/pmc/articles/PMC2886488/ (accessed 24 February 2016).

6. Luther J, Dave M, Higgins PD, Kao JY. Association between Helicobacter pylori infection and inflammatory bowel disease: a meta-analysis and systematic review of the literature. *Inflamm Bowel Dis* 2010;16(6): 1077-84.
   http://www.ncbi.nlm.nih.gov/pubmed/19760778/ (accessed 24 February 2016).

7. Summers RW, Elliott DE, Urban JF Jr, Thompson RA, Weinstock JV. Trichuris suis therapy for active ulcerative colitis: a randomized controlled trial. *Gastroenterology* 2005;128(4): 825-32.
   http://www.ncbi.nlm.nih.gov/pubmed/15825065/ (accessed 24 February 2016).

8. Garg SK, Croft AM, Bager P. Helminth therapy (worms) for induction of remission in inflammatory bowel disease. *Cochrane Database Syst Rev* 2014;1: CD009400.

http://www.ncbi.nlm.nih.gov/pubmed/24442917 (accessed 24 February 2016).

9. Bernstein CN, Rawsthorne P, Cheang M, Blanchard JF. A population-based case control study of potential risk factors for IBD. *Am J Gastroenterol* 2006;101(5): 993-1002. http://www.ncbi.nlm.nih.gov/pubmed/16696783/ (accessed 24 February 2016).

10. Baron S, Turck D, Leplat C, Merle V, Gower-Rousseau C, Marti R, Yzet T, Lerebours E, Dupas JL, Debeugny S, Salomez JL, Cortot A, Colombel JF. Environmental risk factors in paediatric inflammatory bowel diseases: a population based case control study. *Gut* 2005;54(3): 357-63. http://www.ncbi.nlm.nih.gov/pubmed/15710983/ (accessed 24 February 2016).

11. Hampe J, Heymann K, Krawczak M, Schreiber S. Association of inflammatory bowel disease with indicators for childhood antigen and infection exposure. *Int J Colorectal Dis* 2003;18(5): 413-7. http://www.ncbi.nlm.nih.gov/pubmed/12687394/ (accessed 24 February 2016).

12. Calkins BM. A meta-analysis of the role of smoking in inflammatory bowel disease. *Dig Dis Sci* 1989;34(12): 1841-54. http://www.ncbi.nlm.nih.gov/pubmed/2598752 (accessed 24 February 2016).

13. Rubin DT, Hanauer SB. Smoking and inflammatory bowel disease. *Eur J Gastroenterol Hepatol* 2000;12(8): 855-62. http://www.ncbi.nlm.nih.gov/pubmed/10958212 (accessed 24 February 2016).

14. Shields M. Smoking bans: influence on smoking prevalence. *Health Rep* 2007;18(3): 9-24. http://www.ncbi.nlm.nih.gov/pubmed/17892249 (accessed 24 February 2016).

15. Joossens M, Huys G, Cnockaert M, De Preter V, Verbeke K, Rutgeerts P, Vandamme P, Vermeire S. Dysbiosis of the faecal microbiota in patients with Crohn's disease and their unaffected relatives. *Gut* 2011;60(5): 631-7. http://www.ncbi.nlm.nih.gov/pubmed/21209126 (accessed 24 February 2016).

16. Koloski NA, Bret L, Radford-Smith G. Hygiene hypothesis in inflammatory bowel disease: a critical review of the literature. *World J Gastroenterol* 2008;14(2): 165-73.

http://www.ncbi.nlm.nih.gov/pubmed/18186549/ (accessed 24 February 2016).

17. Russel MG, Engels LG, Muris JW, Limonard CB, Volovics A, Brummer RJ, Stockbrügger RW. 'Modern life' in the epidemiology of inflammatory bowel disease: a case-control study with special emphasis on nutritional factors. *Eur J Gastroenterol Hepatol* 1998;10(3): 243-9. http://www.ncbi.nlm.nih.gov/pubmed/9585029/ (accessed 24 February 2016).

18. Amre DK, D'Souza S, Morgan K, Seidman G, Lambrette P, Grimard G, Israel D, Mack D, Ghadirian P, Deslandres C, Chotard V, Budai B, Law L, Levy E, Seidman EG. Imbalances in dietary consumption of fatty acids, vegetables, and fruits are associated with risk for Crohn's disease in children. *Am J Gastroenterol* 2007;102(9): 2016-25. http://www.ncbi.nlm.nih.gov/pubmed/17617201/ (accessed 24 February 2016).

19. Hildebrand H, Malmborg P, Askling J, Ekbom A, Montgomery SM. Early-life exposures associated with antibiotic use and risk of subsequent Crohn's disease. *Scand J Gastroenterol* 2008;43(8): 961-6. http://www.ncbi.nlm.nih.gov/pubmed/19086166/ (accessed 24 February 2016).

20. Hviid A, Svanström H, Frisch M. Antibiotic use and inflammatory bowel diseases in childhood. *Gut* 2011;60(1): 49-54. http://www.ncbi.nlm.nih.gov/pubmed/20966024/ (accessed 24 February 2016).

21. Ananthakrishnan AN, Higuchi LM, Huang ES, Khalili H, Richter JM, Fuchs CS, Chan AT. Aspirin, nonsteroidal anti-inflammatory drug use, and risk for Crohn disease ulcerative colitis. *Ann Intern Med* 2012; 156(5): 350–359. http://www.ncbi.nlm.nih.gov/pmc/articles/PMC3369539/ (accessed 24 February 2016).

22. Kaplan GG, Hubbard J, Korzenik J, Sands BE, Panaccione R, Ghosh S, Wheeler AJ, Villeneuve PJ. The inflammatory bowel diseases and ambient air pollution: a novel association. *Am J Gastroenterol* 2010; 105(11): 2412–2419. http://www.ncbi.nlm.nih.gov/pmc/articles/PMC3180712/ (accessed 24 February 2016).

23. Ananthakrishnan AN, McGinley EL, Binion DG, Saeian K. Ambient air pollution correlates with hospitalizations for inflammatory bowel disease: an ecologic analysis. *Inflamm Bowel Dis* 2011;17(5): 1138-45.

http://www.ncbi.nlm.nih.gov/pubmed/20806342/ (accessed 24 February 2016).

24. Loftus EV Jr. Clinical epidemiology of inflammatory bowel disease: Incidence, prevalence, and environmental influences. *Gastroenterology* 2004;126(6): 1504-17.
   http://www.ncbi.nlm.nih.gov/pubmed/15168363/ (accessed 24 February 2016).

25. Khalili H, Huang ES, Ananthakrishnan AN, Higuchi L, Richter JM, Fuchs CS, Chan AT. Geographical variation and incidence of inflammatory bowel disease among US women. *Gut* 2012; 61(12): 1686–1692.
   http://www.ncbi.nlm.nih.gov/pmc/articles/PMC3418414/ (accessed 24 February 2016).This leaflet is not available on the Core website any more
   http://www.corecharity.org.uk/conditions/ulcerative-colitis

26. Crohn's & Colitis UK. What is ulcerative colitis? *Crohn's & Colitis UK*. November 2013.
   http://www.crohnsandcolitis.org.uk/Resources/CrohnsAndColitisUK/Documents/Publications/Booklets/Ulcerative-Colitis.pdf (accessed 24 February 2016).

27. Core. *Information about Crohn's Disease*. Core. 2014.
   http://beta.corecharity.org.uk/wp-content/uploads/2015/10/Core-Patient-Information-Crohns-Disease.pdf (accessed 24 February 2016).

28. Core. *Information about Crohn's Disease*. Core. 2014.
   http://beta.corecharity.org.uk/wp-content/uploads/2015/10/Core-Patient-Information-Crohns-Disease.pdf (accessed 24 February 2016).

29. Core. *Information about Crohn's Disease*. Core. 2014.
   http://beta.corecharity.org.uk/wp-content/uploads/2015/10/Core-Patient-Information-Crohns-Disease.pdf (accessed 24 February 2016).

30. Crohn's & Colitis UK. *What is ulcerative colitis?* Crohn's & Colitis UK. November 2013.
   http://www.crohnsandcolitis.org.uk/Resources/CrohnsAndColitisUK/Documents/Publications/Booklets/Ulcerative-Colitis.pdf (accessed 24 February 2016).

31. Crohn's & Colitis UK. *Drugs used in IBD*. Edition 5. March 2014. Crohn's & Colitis UK.
   http://s3-eu-west-1.amazonaws.com/files.crohnsandcolitis.org.uk/Publications/drugs-used-in-IBD.pdf (accessed 24 February 2016).

32. Crohn's & Colitis UK. *Drugs used in IBD*. Edition 5. March 2014. Crohn's & Colitis UK. http://s3-eu-west-1.amazonaws.com/files.crohnsandcolitis.org.uk/Publications/drugs-used-in-IBD.pdf (accessed 24 February 2016).

33. Crohn's & Colitis UK. *What is ulcerative colitis?* Crohn's & Colitis UK. November 2013. http://www.crohnsandcolitis.org.uk/Resources/CrohnsAndColitisUK/Documents/Publications/Booklets/Ulcerative-Colitis.pdf (accessed 24 February 2016).

34. Crohn's & Colitis UK. *What is ulcerative colitis?* Crohn's & Colitis UK. November 2013. http://www.crohnsandcolitis.org.uk/Resources/CrohnsAndColitisUK/Documents/Publications/Booklets/Ulcerative-Colitis.pdf (accessed 24 February 2016).

35. Core. *Information about Crohn's Disease*. Core. 2014. http://beta.corecharity.org.uk/wp-content/uploads/2015/10/Core-Patient-Information-Crohns-Disease.pdf (accessed 24 February 2016).

36. NHS Choices. Crohn's disease – treatment. *NHS Choices*. 17 April 2015. http://www.nhs.uk/Conditions/Crohns-disease/Pages/Treatment.aspx (accessed 24 February 2016).

37. NHS Crohn's Disease. www.nhs.uk/Conditions/Crohns-disease/Pages/Treatment.aspx (accessed 5 July 2016).

38. Ghouri YA, Richards DM, Rahimi EF, Krill JT, Jelinek KA, DuPont AW. Systematic review of randomized controlled trials of probiotics, prebiotics, and synbiotics in inflammatory bowel disease. *Clin Exp Gastroenterol* 2014; 7: 473–487. http://www.ncbi.nlm.nih.gov/pmc/articles/PMC4266241/ (accessed 24 February 2016).

39. Ghouri YA, Richards DM, Rahimi EF, Krill JT, Jelinek KA, DuPont AW. Systematic review of randomized controlled trials of probiotics, prebiotics, and synbiotics in inflammatory bowel disease. *Clin Exp Gastroenterol* 2014; 7: 473–487. http://www.ncbi.nlm.nih.gov/pmc/articles/PMC4266241/ (accessed 24 February 2016).

40. Ruben J et al. Faecal microbiota transportation as therapy for IBD: a systematic review and meta analysis. *Journal of Crohn's and Colitits* 2014; 8(12): 1569-1581.

41. Lewis JD. The role of diet in inflammatory bowel disease. *Gastroenterology and Hepatology* 2016; 12(1): 51-53.

Chapter 7

1. Beating bowel cancer. Facts and figures. *Beating Bowel Cancer*. 18 May 2015.
   https://www.beatingbowelcancer.org/facts-and-figures (accessed 18 March 2016).

2. Cancer Research UK. Statistics and outlook for bowel cancer. *Cancer Research UK*. 26 August 2015.
   http://www.cancerresearchuk.org/about-cancer/type/bowel-cancer/treatment/statistics-and-outlook-for-bowel-cancer (accessed 24 February 2016).

3. Cancer Research UK. Survival statistics for bowel cancer. *Cancer Research UK*. 26 August 2015.
   http://www.cancerresearchuk.org/about-cancer/type/bowel-cancer/treatment/statistics-and-outlook-for-bowel-cancer (accessed 1 August 2016).

4. Center MM, Jemal A, Ward E. International trends in colorectal cancer incidence rates. *Cancer Epidemiol Biomarkers Prev* 2009; 18: 1688
   http://cebp.aacrjournals.org/content/18/6/1688 (accessed 24 February 2016).

5. World Cancer Research Fund International. Colorectal cancer statistics. *World Cancer Research Fund International*. 2014.
   http://www.wcrf.org/int/cancer-facts-figures/data-specific-cancers/colorectal-cancer-statistics (accessed 18 March 2016).

6. Beating bowel cancer. Facts and figures. *Beating Bowel Cancer*. 18 May 2015.
   https://www.beatingbowelcancer.org/facts-and-figures (accessed 18 March 2016).

7. UEG. Incidence of colorectal cancer increasing in young people: family doctors urged to be on the alert for alarm symptoms. *United European Gastroenterology*. 24 March 2015.
   https://www.ueg.eu/press/releases/ueg-press-release/article/incidence-of-colorectal-cancer-increasing-in-young-people-family-doctors-urged-to-be-on-the-alert-f/ (accessed 24 February 2016).

8. Cancer Research UK. Bowel cancer risk factors overview. *Cancer Research UK*. 11February 2015.
   http://www.cancerresearchuk.org/health-professional/cancer-statistics/statistics-by-cancer-type/bowel-cancer/risk-factors#heading-Zero (accessed 24 February 2016).

9. NHS Choices. Red meat and the risk of bowel cancer. *NHS Choices*. 4 March 2015.

http://www.nhs.uk/Livewell/Goodfood/Pages/red-meat.aspx (accessed 24 February 2016).

10. Scientific Advisory Committee on Nutrition. *SACN Iron and health report*. Public Health England. 25 February 2011. https://www.gov.uk/government/publications/sacn-iron-and-health-report (accessed 24 February 2016).

11. Hewitson P, Glasziou PP, Irwig L, Towler B, Watson E. Screening for colorectal cancer using the faecal occult blood test, Hemoccult. *Cochrane*. 24 January 2007. http://www.cochrane.org/CD001216/COLOCA_screening-for-colorectal-cancer-using-the-faecal-occult-blood-test-hemoccult (accessed 24 May 2016).

12. Gov.uk. Bowel cancer screening: commission, provide, inform. *Public Health England* 1 January 2015. http://www.cancerscreening.nhs.uk/bowel/publications/bowel-cancer-the-facts.pdf (accessed 24 May 2016).

13. Cancer Research UK. Stomach cancer survival statistics. *Cancer Research UK*. 10 December 2014. http://www.cancerresearchuk.org/health-professional/cancer-statistics/statistics-by-cancer-type/stomach-cancer/survival#heading-Zero (accessed 24 February 2016).

14. American Cancer Society. *Cancer facts & figures 2015*. American Cancer Society. 2015. http://www.cancer.org/acs/groups/content/@editorial/documents/document/acspc-044552.pdf (accessed 24 February 2016).

15. Wroblewski LE, Peek RM Jr, Wilson KT. Helicobacter pylori and gastric cancer: factors that modulate disease risk. *Clin Microbiol Rev* 2010; 23(4): 713-39. http://www.ncbi.nlm.nih.gov/pubmed/20930071 (accessed 24 May 2016).

16. Ren JS, Kamangar F, Forman D, Islami F. Pickled food and risk of gastric cancer--a systematic review and meta-analysis of English and Chinese literature. *Cancer Epidemiol Biomarkers Prev* 2012 Jun;21(6): 905-15. http://www.ncbi.nlm.nih.gov/pubmed/22499775 (accessed 24 February 2016).

17. Zhang Y. Epidemiology of esophageal cancer. *World J Gastroenterol* 2013; 19(34): 5598–5606. http://www.ncbi.nlm.nih.gov/pmc/articles/PMC3769895/ (accessed 24 February 2016).

18. Zhang Y. Epidemiology of esophageal cancer. *World J Gastroenterol* 2013; 19(34): 5598–5606.
     http://www.ncbi.nlm.nih.gov/pmc/articles/PMC3769895/ (accessed 25 February 2016).

19. WCRF. Reducing your risk of oesophageal cancer. *World Cancer Research Fund*. October 2013.
     http://www.wcrf-uk.org/uk/preventing-cancer/cancer-types/reducing-your-risk-oesophageal-cancer (accessed 25 February 2016).

20. Castellsagué X, Muñoz N, De Stefani E, Victora CG, Castelletto R, Rolón PA, Quintana MJ. Independent and joint effects of tobacco smoking and alcohol drinking on the risk of esophageal cancer in men and women. *International Journal of Cancer* 1999; 82(5): 657–664.
     http://onlinelibrary.wiley.com/doi/10.1002/%28SICI%291097-0215%2819990827%2982:5%3C657::AID-IJC7%3E3.0.CO;2-C/full (accessed 25 February 2016).

21. Zhang Y. Epidemiology of esophageal cancer. *World J Gastroenterol* 2013; 19(34): 5598–5606.
     http://www.ncbi.nlm.nih.gov/pmc/articles/PMC3769895/ (accessed 24 February 2016).

22. NHS Choices. Oesophageal cancer – causes. *NHS Choices*. 30 June 2014.
     http://www.nhs.uk/Conditions/Cancer-of-the-oesophagus/Pages/Causes.aspx (accessed 25 February 2016).

23. Zhang Y. Epidemiology of esophageal cancer. *World J Gastroenterol* 2013; 19(34): 5598–5606.
     http://www.ncbi.nlm.nih.gov/pmc/articles/PMC3769895/ (accessed 25 February 2016).

24. NHS Choices. Oesophageal cancer – causes. *NHS Choices*. 30 June 2014.
     http://www.nhs.uk/Conditions/Cancer-of-the-oesophagus/Pages/Causes.aspx (accessed 24 February 2016).

25. Islami F, Boffetta P, Ren J, Pedoeim L, Khatib D, Kamangar F. High-temperature beverages and foods and esophageal cancer risk - A systematic review. *Int J Cancer* 2009; 125(3): 491–524.
     http://www.ncbi.nlm.nih.gov/pmc/articles/PMC2773211/ (accessed 25 February 2016).

26. NHS Choices. Oesophageal cancer – causes. *NHS Choices*. 30 June 2014.
     http://www.nhs.uk/Conditions/Cancer-of-the-oesophagus/Pages/Causes.aspx (accessed 25 February 2016).

27. NICE. *Suspected cancer: recognition and referral*. NICE guidelines [NG12]. June 2015.
     https://www.nice.org.uk/guidance/ng12/chapter/1-

Recommendations-organised-by-site-of-cancer#upper-gastrointestinal-tract-cancers (accessed 25 February 2016).

28. Cancer Research UK. Statistics and outlook for oesophageal cancer. *Cancer Research UK*. 17 June 2015. http://www.cancerresearchuk.org/about-cancer/type/oesophageal-cancer/treatment/statistics-and-outlook-for-oesophageal-cancer (accessed 25 February 2016).

29. Cancer Research UK. Statistics and outlook for oesophageal cancer. *Cancer Research UK*. 17 June 2015. http://www.cancerresearchuk.org/about-cancer/type/oesophageal-cancer/treatment/statistics-and-outlook-for-oesophageal-cancer (accessed 25 February 2016).

30. Cancer Research UK. Symptoms of gallbladder cancer. *Cancer Research UK*. 6 June 2014 http://www.cancerresearchuk.org/about-cancer/type/gallbladder-cancer/about/symptoms-of-gallbladder-cancer (accessed 24 May 2016).

31. Cancer Research UK. Which surgery for gallbladder cancer? *Cancer Research UK*. 18 June 2014. http://www.cancerresearchuk.org/about-cancer/type/gallbladder-cancer/treatment/surgery/which-surgery-for-gallbladder-cancer (accessed 25 February 2016).

32. Reducing your risk of gallbladder cancer. www.wcrf-uk.org/uk/preventing-cancer/cancer-types/reducing-your-risk-gallbladder (accessed 5 July 2016).

33. Pancreatic Cancer Action. Pancreatic cancer symptoms. *Pancreatic Cancer Action*. 3 January 2014. https://pancreaticcanceraction.org/about-pancreatic-cancer/symptoms/ (accessed 25 February 2016).

34. Cancer Research UK. Statistics and outlook for pancreatic cancer. *Cancer Research UK*. 17 June 2015. http://www.cancerresearchuk.org/about-cancer/type/pancreatic-cancer/treatment/statistics-and-outlook-for-pancreatic-cancer (accessed 25 February 2016).

35. NICE. *Suspected cancer: recognition and referral*. NICE guidelines [NG12]. June 2015. https://www.nice.org.uk/guidance/ng12/chapter/1-Recommendations-organised-by-site-of-cancer#lung-and-pleural-cancers (accessed 25 February 2016).

36. Paddock C. Blood test for early stage pancreatic cancer looks promising. *Medical News Today*. 25 June 2015.

http://www.medicalnewstoday.com/articles/295862.php
(accessed 25 February 2016).

37. Whiteman H. Urine test for pancreatic cancer a step closer. *Medical News Today*. 3 August 2015.
http://www.medicalnewstoday.com/articles/297621.php
(accessed 25 February 2016).

38. Medical News Today. Pancreatic cancer: researchers develop a new therapy concept. *Medical News Today*. 25 September 2015.
http://www.medicalnewstoday.com/releases/299971.php
(accessed 24 February 2016).

39. Cancer Research UK. Kidney cancer. *Cancer Research UK*. 24 February 2016.
http://www.cancerresearchuk.org/about-cancer/type/kidney-cancer/ (accessed 25 February 2016).

40. Liang S, Lv G, Chen W, Jiang J, Wang J. Height and kidney cancer risk: a meta-analysis of prospective studies. *J Cancer Res Clin Oncol* 2015;141(10): 1799-807.
http://www.ncbi.nlm.nih.gov/pubmed/25388591 (accessed 25 February 2016).

41. Target Ovarian Cancer. Ovarian Cancer Symptoms. *Target Ovarian Cancer*. January 2015.
http://www.targetovariancancer.org.uk/about-ovarian-cancer/what-ovarian-cancer/ovarian-cancer-symptoms?section=78&sectiontitle= (accessed 25 February 2016).

42. Target Ovarian Cancer. Ovarian Cancer Symptoms. *Target Ovarian Cancer*. January 2015.
http://www.targetovariancancer.org.uk/about-ovarian-cancer/what-ovarian-cancer/ovarian-cancer-symptoms?section=78&sectiontitle= (accessed 25 February 2016).

43. WCRF. Reducing your risk of ovarian cancer. *World Cancer Research Fund*. March 2014.
http://www.wcrf-uk.org/uk/preventing-cancer/cancer-types/reducing-your-risk-ovarian-cancer (accessed 25 February 2016).

44. Macmillan Cancer Support. Living with or beyond cancer. *Macmillan Cancer Support*. 2016.
http://www.macmillan.org.uk/GetInvolved/Campaigns/Weareaforceforchange/Survivorship/Livingwithorbeyondcancer.aspx (accessed 25 February 2016).

45. Macmillan Cancer Support. *Guidance: The Practical Management of the Gastrointestinal Symptoms of Pelvic Radiation Disease*. Macmillan Cancer Support. 2014.

http://www.macmillan.org.uk/Documents/AboutUs/
Health_professionals/P215TRMGIBooklet_AW.pdf (accessed 25
February 2016).

46. PRDA. What is pelvic radiation disease. *Pelvic Radiation Disease
Association*. Nd.
http://www.prda.org.uk/what-pelvic-radiation-disease (accessed
25 February 2016).

47. Macmillan Cancer Support. *Guidance: The Practical Management of
the Gastrointestinal Symptoms of Pelvic Radiation Disease*. Macmillan
Cancer Support. 2014.
http://www.macmillan.org.uk/Documents/AboutUs/
Health_professionals/P215TRMGIBooklet_AW.pdf (accessed 25
February 2016).

Chapter 8

1. Neal G. Symptomatolgy of gastrointestinal disease. In: Warrell DA, Cox TM, Firth JD (Eds) *Oxford Textbook of Medicine* 5th edition. Oxford, UK: Oxford University Press; 2010: 2205-2209.

2. NICE. Dyspepsia - proven GORD. NICE. November 2012. http://cks.nice.org.uk/dyspepsia-proven-gord#!backgroundsub (Accessed 1 August 2016).

3. British Society of Gastroenterology. Dyspepsia management guidelines. British Society of Gastroenterology, 2002. www.bsg.org.uk (Accessed 25 February 2016).

4. National Collaborating Centre for Cancer (2015) *Suspected cancer: recognition and referral. Full guideline June 2015.* National Institute for Health and Care Excellence. www.nice.org.uk mentioned on NICE. Clinical Knowledge Summary: Dyspepsia – proven GORD. November 2012.http://cks.nice.org.uk/dyspepsia-proven-gord#!scenario (Accessed 24 May 2016).

5. BMJ Group. GORD in adults. London, UK: BMJ Publishing Group Limited; 2015. besthealth-bmj.com/pdf/392764.pdf (Accessed 1 August 2016).

6. Dent J, El-Serag HB, Wallander M-A, Johansson S. Epidemiology of gastro-oesophageal reflux disease: a systematic review. *Gut* 2005; 54(5): 710–717.

7. NICE. Scenario: Dyspepsia – proven gastro-oesophageal reflux disease. NICE. November 2012. http://cks.nice.org.uk/dyspepsia-proven-gord#!scenario (Accessed 25 February 2016).

8. Hershcovici T et al. Pharmacological management of GERD; where does it stand now? *Trends in Pharmacological Science* 2010; 32(4): 258-264.

9. Macmillan Cancer Support. Barrett's oesophagus. 30 April 2014. http://www.macmillan.org.uk/information-and-support/diagnosing/causes-and-risk-factors/pre-cancerous-conditions/barretts-oesophagus.html (Accessed 1 August 2016)

10. NHS Choices. Hearburn and gastro-oesophageal reflux disease (GORD) – complications. http://www.nhs.uk/Conditions/Gastroesophageal-reflux-disease/Pages/Complications.aspx (Accessed 1 August 2016)

10A. Cancer Research UK. Barrett's oesophagus. http://www.cancerresearchuk.org/about-cancer/cancers-in-general/cancer-questions/what-is-barretts-oesophagus

11. Patient. Globus sensation. *Patient* 27 July 2015. http://patient.

info/health/globus-sensation-leaflet (Accessed 1 August 2016)

12. Guy's and St Thomas'NHS Foundation Trust. Globus. NHS. December 2012. http://www.guysandstthomas.nhs.uk/ resources/patientinformation/therapies/slt/Globus.pdf (Accessed 1 August 2016).

13. Levitt M, Modi R. Belching, bloating and flatulence. *American College of Gastroenterology* 2004, updated 2013. http://patients. gi.org/topics/belching-bloating-and-flatulence/ (Accessed 1 August 2016).

14. Mayo Clinic. Bloating, belching and intestinal gas: How to avoid them. Mayo Clinic. 15 April 2014. http://www.mayoclinic.org/ diseases-conditions/gas-and-gaspains/in-depth/gas-and-gas-pains/art-20044739 (Accessed 1 August 2016).

15. Core. Peptic ulcers. http://www.corecharity.org.uk/conditions/ peptic-ulcers (Accessed 25 February 2016).

16. NHS Choices. Stomach ulcer – symptoms. NHS Choices. 21 May 2015. http://www.nhs.uk/Conditions/Peptic-ulcer/Pages/ Symptoms.aspx (Accessed 1 August 2016).

17. Ahmed N. 23 years after the discovery of Helicobacter pylori: Is the debate over? *Ann Clin Microbiol Antimicrob* 2005; 4: 17.

18. NHS Choices. Stomach ulcer – symptoms. NHS Choices. 21 May 2015. http://www.nhs.uk/conditions/peptic-ulcer/Pages/ Introduction.aspx (Accessed 1 August 2016).

19. Marshall BJ, Warren JR. Unidentified curved bacilli in the stomach of patients with gastritis and peptic ulceration. *Lancet* 1984; 1(8390): 1311-1315.

20. NHS Choices. Stomach ulcer – symptoms. *NHS Choices* 21 May 2015. http://www.nhs.uk/Conditions/Peptic-ulcer/Pages/ Symptoms.aspx (Accessed 25 February 2016).

21. Milosavljevic T, Kostić-Milosavljević M, Jovanović I, Krstić M. Complications of peptic ulcer disease. *Digestive Disease* 2011; 29(5): 491-493.

21A. Core. Gallstones. 2014. Corecharity.org.uk/gut-and-liver-and-pancreas/liver/gallstones/ (Accessed 1 August 2016).

22. Snowden FM. Emerging and reemerging diseases: a historical perspective. *Immunological Reviews: Special Issue: Immunology of Emerging Infections* 2008; 225(1): 9–26. doi: 10.1111/j.1600-065X.2008.00677

22A. Shaffer EA. Epidemiology and risk factors for gallstone disease: has the paradigm changed in the 21st century? *Curr Gastroenterol Rep* 2005; 7(2): 132-140.

23. Shaheen NJ, Hansen RA, Morgan DR, Gangarosa LM, Ringel Y, Thiny MT, Russo MW, Sandler RS. The burden of gastrointestinal and liver diseases, 2006. *American Journal of Gastroenterology* 2006; 101(9): 2128-2138.

24. Stinton LM, Shaffer EA. Epidemiology of gallbladder disease: cholelithiasis and cancer. *Gut & Liver* 2012; 6(2): 172–187.

25. Shaffer EA. Epidemiology and risk factors for gallstone disease: has the paradigm changed in the 21st century? *Curr Gastroenterol Rep* 2005; 7(2): 132-40.

26. Stinton LM, Shaffer EA. Edidemiology of gallbladder disease; cholelithiasis and cancer. *Gut Liver* 2012; 6(2): 172-187.

27. Shaffer EA. Epidemiology and risk factors for gallstone disease: has the paradigm changed in the 21st century? *Curr Gastroenterol Rep* 2005; 7(2): 132-140.

28. Sarin SK, Negi VS, Dewan R, Sasan S et al. High familial prevalence of gallstones in the first degree relatives of gallstone patients. *Hepatology* 1995; 22(1): 138-141.

29. Sarin SK, Negi VS, Dewan R, Sasan S et al. High familial prevalence of gallstones in the first degree relatives of gallstone patients. *Hepatology* 1995; 22(1): 138-141.

30. Expert Panel on Detection, Evaluation, and Treatment of High Blood Cholesterol in Adults. Executive Summary of the Third Report of the National Cholesterol Education Program (NCEP) Expert Panel on Detection, Evaluation, and Treatment of High Blood Cholesterol in Adults (Adult Treatment Panel III). *JAMA* 2001; 285(19): 2486-2497.

31. Li VK, Pulido N, Fajnwaks P, Szomstein S, Rosenthal R, Martinez-Duartez P. Predictors of gallstone formation after bariatric surgery: a multivariate analysis of risk factors comparing gastric bypass, gastric banding, and sleeve gastrectomy. *Surg Endosc* 2009; 23(7): 1640-1644.

32. Everhart JE. Contributions of obesity and weight loss to gallstone disease. *Annals of Internal Medicine* 1993; 119(10): 1029-1035.

33. Wudel LJ Jr, Wright JK, Debelak JP, Allos TM, Shyr Y, Chapman WCJ. Prevention of gallstone formation in morbidly obese patients undergoing rapid weight loss: results of a randomized controlled pilot study. *Surgical Research* 2002; 102(1): 50-56.

34. Li VK, Pulido N, Fajnwaks P, Szomstein S, Rosenthal R, Martinez-Duartez P. Predictors of gallstone formation after bariatric surgery: a multivariate analysis of risk factors comparing gastric bypass, gastric banding, and sleeve gastrectomy. *Surg Endosc* 2009; 23(7): 1640-1644.

35. Lee DW, Gilmore CJ, Bonorris G, Cohen H, Marks JW, Cho-Sue M, Meiselman MS, Schoenfield LJ.Effect of dietary cholesterol on biliary lipids in patients with gallstones and normal subjects. *American Journal of Clinical Nutrition* 1985; 42(3): 414-420.

36. Tsai CJ, Leitzmann MF, Willett WC, Giovannucci EL. Long-chain saturated fatty acids consumption and risk of gallstone disease among men. *Annals of Surgery* 2008; 247(1): 95-103.

37. Scragg RK, McMichael AJ, Baghurst PA Diet, alcohol, and relative weight in gall stone disease: a case-control study. *British Medical Journal (Clinical Research Edition)* 1984; 288(6424): 1113-1119.

38. Stinton LM, Shaffer EA. Edidemiology of gallbladder disease; cholelithiasis and cancer. *Gut Liver* 2012; 6(2): 172-187.

Chapter 9

1. Longstreth GF, Thompson WG, Chey WD, Houghton LA, Mearin F, Spiller RC. Functional bowel disorders. *Gastroenterology* 2006;130(5): 1480-91.http://www.ncbi.nlm.nih.gov/pubmed/16678561 (accessed 25 February 2016).

2. NICE. Constipation. *NICE*. October 2015. http://cks.nice.org.uk/constipation#!backgroundsub (accessed 25 February 2016).

3. Pinto Sanchez MI and Bercik P. Epidemiology and burden of chronic constipation. *Can J Gastroenterol* 2011; 25(Suppl B): 11B–15B. http://www.ncbi.nlm.nih.gov/pmc/articles/PMC3206560/ (accessed 24 May 2016).

4. American College of Gastroenterology Chronic Constipation Task Force. An evidence-based approach to the management of chronic constipation in North America. *Am J Gastroenterol</ital.* 2005;100 Suppl 1: S1-4. http://www.ncbi.nlm.nih.gov/pubmed/16008640 (accessed 25 February 2016).

5. Pare P, Ferrazzi S, Thompson WG, Irvine EJ and Rance L. An epidemiological survey of constipation in Canada: definitions, rates, demographics, and predictors of health care seeking. *Am J Gastroenterol* 2001; 96, 3130–3137.

6. NHS Choices. Constipation. *NHS Choices* 24 December 2015. http://www.nhs.uk/Conditions/Constipation/Pages/Introduction.aspx (accessed 24 May 2016).

7. HSCIC. Prescriptions Dispensed in the Community, Statistics for England – 2000-2010 [NS]. *HSCIC*. 27 July 2011. http://www.hscic.gov.uk/searchcatalogue?productid=228&q=title%3a%22Prescriptions+Dispensed+in+the+Community%2c+Statistics+for+England%22&sort=Relevance&size=10&page=1#top (accessed 25 February 2016).

8. HSCIC. *Prescription Cost Analysis England 2015*. HSCIC. 7 April 2016. http://www.hscic.gov.uk/catalogue/PUB20200/pres-cost-anal-eng-2015-rep.pdf (accessed 24 May 2016).

9. NICE. Constipation. *NICE*. October 2015. http://cks.nice.org.uk/constipation#!backgroundsub:8 (accessed 25 February 2016).

10. Gallegos-Orozco JF, Foxx-Orenstein AE, Sterler SM, Stoa JM. Chronic constipation in the elderly. *Am J Gastroenterol* 2012;107(1): 18-25.

http://www.ncbi.nlm.nih.gov/pubmed/21989145/ (accessed 25 February 2016).

11. Gallegos-Orozco JF, Foxx-Orenstein AE, Sterler SM, Stoa JM. Chronic constipation in the elderly. *Am J Gastroenterol* 2012 ;107(1): 18-25.
    http://www.ncbi.nlm.nih.gov/pubmed/21989145/ (accessed 25 February 2016).

12. Cullen G, O'Donoghue D. Constipation and pregnancy. *Best Pract Res Clin Gastroenterol* 2007;21(5): 807-18.
    http://www.ncbi.nlm.nih.gov/pubmed/17889809 (accessed 25 February 2016).

13. NHS Choices. Constipation. *NHS Choices*. 24 December 2015.
    http://www.nhs.uk/Conditions/Constipation/Pages/Introduction.aspx (accessed 25 February 2016).

14. NICE. Constipation. *NICE*. October 2015.
    http://cks.nice.org.uk/constipation#!backgroundsub:11 (accessed 25 February 2016).

15. American College of Gastroenterology Chronic Constipation Task Force. An evidence-based approach to the management of chronic constipation in North America. *Am J Gastroenterol* 2005;100 Suppl 1: S1-4.
    http://www.ncbi.nlm.nih.gov/pubmed/16008640 (accessed 25 February 2016).

16. NHS Choices. Constipation – treatment. *NHS Choices*. 24 December 2015.
    http://www.nhs.uk/Conditions/Constipation/Pages/Treatment.aspx (accessed 25 February 2016).

17. NICE. Constipation. *NICE*. October 2015.
    http://cks.nice.org.uk/constipation#!topicsummary (accessed 25 February 2016).

18. NICE. Constipation: Factors affecting choice of laxative. *NICE*. October 2015.
    http://cks.nice.org.uk/constipation#!prescribinginfosub:2 (accessed 25 February 2016).

19. NICE. Constipation: Scenario: Adults. *NICE*. October 2015.
    http://cks.nice.org.uk/constipation#!scenario (accessed 25 February 2016).

20. NICE. Constipation: Factors affecting choice of laxative. *NICE*. October 2015.
    http://cks.nice.org.uk/constipation#!prescribinginfosub:2 (accessed 25 February 2016).

21. NICE. Lubiprostone for treating chronic idiopathic constipation. *NICE technology appraisal guidance* [TA318]. July 2014. https://www.nice.org.uk/guidance/ta318 (accessed 25 February 2016).

22. NICE. Haemorrhoids. *NICE*. September 2012. http://cks.nice.org.uk/haemorrhoids#!topicsummary (accessed 25 February 2016).

23. Johanson JF, Sonnenberg A. The prevalence of hemorrhoids and chronic constipation. An epidemiologic study. *Gastroenterology* 1990;98(2): 380-6. http://www.ncbi.nlm.nih.gov/pubmed/2295392 (accessed 25 February 2016).

24. Johanson JF, Sonnenberg A. The prevalence of hemorrhoids and chronic constipation. An epidemiologic study. *Gastroenterology* 1990;98(2): 380-6. http://www.ncbi.nlm.nih.gov/pubmed/2295392 (accessed 25 February 2016).

25. NICE. Suspected cancers: recognition and referral. *NICE guidelines* [NG12]. June 2015. https://www.nice.org.uk/guidance/ng12/chapter/1-recommendations-organised-by-site-of-cancer#lower-gastrointestinal-tract-cancers (accessed 1 August 2016).

26. NICE. Haemorrhoids (piles) - Surgery. NICE. March 2016. http://www.nhs.uk/Conditions/Haemorrhoids/Pages/Surgery.aspx (Accessed 14 August 2016).

27. NICE. Anal fissure. *NICE*. November 2012. http://cks.nice.org.uk/anal-fissure (accessed 25 February 2016).

28. Core. *Information about Diverticular disease*. Core. 2014. http://beta.corecharity.org.uk/wp-content/uploads/2015/10/Core-Patient-Information-Diverticular-Disease.pdf (accessed 25 February 2016).

29. Aldoori WH, Giovannucci EL, Rimm EB, Wing AL, Trichopoulos DV, Willett WC. A prospective study of diet and the risk of symptomatic diverticular disease in men. *Am J Clin Nutr* 1994;60(5): 757-764. http://ajcn.nutrition.org/content/60/5/757.abstract?ijkey=cce37418fc148fbe809c801bc2d7962b9d077aab&keytype2=tf_ipsecsha (accessed 25 February 2016).

30. Crowe FL, Appleby PN, Allen NE, J Key TJ. Diet and risk of diverticular disease in Oxford cohort of European Prospective Investigation into Cancer and Nutrition (EPIC): prospective study

of British vegetarians and non-vegetarians. *BMJ* 2011;343.
http://www.bmj.com/content/343/bmj.d4131.abstract?ijkey=cd4
990578316903767d0c69f41d6821b993dd876&keytype2=tf_ipsecsha
(accessed 25 February 2016).

31. Crowe FL, Appleby PN, Allen NE, J Key TJ. Diet and risk of
diverticular disease in Oxford cohort of European Prospective
Investigation into Cancer and Nutrition (EPIC): prospective study
of British vegetarians and non-vegetarians. *BMJ* 2011;343.
http://www.bmj.com/content/343/bmj.d4131.abstract?ijkey=cd4
990578316903767d0c69f41d6821b993dd876&keytype2=tf_ipsecsha
(accessed 25 February 2016).

32. Crowe FL, Balkwill A, Cairns BJ, Appleby PN, Green J, Reeves
GK, Key TJ, Beral V. Source of dietary fibre and diverticular
disease incidence: a prospective study of UK women. *Gut* 2014;63:
1450-1456.
http://gut.bmj.com/content/63/9/1450.abstract?ijkey=ba3ff4
0dad24946870deedd7da8b0c4601b5744e&keytype2=tf_ipsecsha
(accessed 25 February 2016).

33. Loffeld RJ. Diverticulosis of the colon is rare amongst immigrants
living in the Zaanstreek region in the Netherlands. *Colorectal Dis*
2005;7(6): 559-62.
http://www.ncbi.nlm.nih.gov/pubmed/16232235?dopt=Abstract
(accessed 25 February 2016).

34. Granlund1 J, Svensson T, Olén O, Hjern F, Pedersen NL,
Magnusson PKE, Thelin Schmidt P. The genetic influence on
diverticular disease – a twin study. *Alimentary Pharmacology &
Therapeutics* 2012; 35(9): 1103–1107.
http://onlinelibrary.wiley.com/doi/10.1111/j.1365-
2036.2012.05069.x/full (accessed 25 February 2016).

35. Reichert MC, Lammert F. The genetic epidemiology of
diverticulosis and diverticular disease: Emerging evidence. *United
European Gastroenterology Journal* 2015; 0(0): 1-10.
http://ueg.sagepub.com/content/early/2015/03/05/2050640615
576676.full (accessed 25 February 2016).

Index

Footnote: Abbreviations used: GORD, gastro-oesophageal reflux disease; IBD, inflammatory bowel disease; IBS, irritable bowel syndrome

Footnote: Abbreviations used: GORD, gastro-oesophageal reflux disease; IBD, inflammatory bowel disease; IBS, irritable bowel syndrome

Footnote: Abbreviations used: GORD, gastro-oesophageal reflux disease; IBD, inflammatory bowel disease; IBS, irritable bowel syndrome

Footnote: Abbreviations used: GORD, gastro-oesophageal reflux disease; IBD, inflammatory bowel disease; IBS, irritable bowel syndrome

Footnote: Abbreviations used: GORD, gastro-oesophageal reflux disease; IBD, inflammatory bowel disease; IBS, irritable bowel syndrome

Footnote: Abbreviations used: GORD, gastro-oesophageal reflux disease; IBD, inflammatory bowel disease; IBS, irritable bowel syndrome

Footnote: Abbreviations used: GORD, gastro-oesophageal reflux disease; IBD, inflammatory bowel disease; IBS, irritable bowel syndrome

Notes

Notes

Notes

Notes

Sustainable Medicine

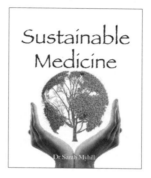

Sustainable Medicine
– whistle-blowing on 21st century medical practice
By Dr Sarah Myhill

Print ISBN: 978-1-78161-032-9
Ebook ISBN: 978-1-78161-033-6

Based on the essential premise that contemporary western medicine is
failing to address the root causes of disease
processes, Sustainable Medicine aims to empower readers to heal
themselves through addressing the underlying causes of
their health problems. Dr Myhill spells out her programme for
maximising health and keeping lifestyle diseases at bay without
recourse to pharmaceuticals.

> **Winner of the People's Book Prize**
> **Best Achievement Award 2016**

Coming soon...

How to feel differently about food

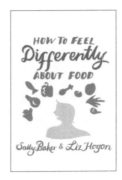

How to Feel Differently About Food
Liberation and Recovery from Emotional Eating
By Sally Baker & Liz Hogon

Print ISBN: 978-1-78161-094-7
Ebook ISBN: 978-1-78161-095-4

How to Feel Differently about Food cuts a clear path through the conflicting nutritional information that fills the popular media to reveal the best way to eat for improved health and enhanced mood, boost energy without triggering feelings of hunger and stop wildly fluctuating blood-sugar levels that lead to cravings. They explain how to make informed and appetising food choices and how to implement small but empowering new eating habits from breakfast onwards. Learning new ways of thinking and feeling about food will naturally enable readers to approach food differently. These positive changes are designed to be effortlessly integrated into a busy life with minimum planning and preparation, including how to eat for nourishment, become healthier, lose excess weight if appropriate, and boost mood as well as help to combat anxiety and depression.

Coming soon...

Inflammatory Bowel Disease

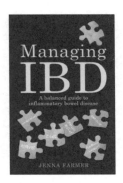

Managing IBD
A balanced guide to inflammatory bowel disease
By Jenna Farmer
With IBD nurse specialist, Kaye Downes,
and counsellor/therapist, Sally Baker

Print ISBN: 978-1-78161-098-5
Ebook ISBN: 978-1-78161-099-2

Jenna Farmer offers an holistic and positive guide to living with IBD, combining conventional, nutritional, stress reduction and other lifestyle approaches, drawing on her blogs, ebooks and website www. abalancedbelly.co.uk. Throughout, the book is 'illustrated' with case histories from Jenna's blog and other contacts, and from her own experience of delayed diagnosis and listening to her symptoms.

Irritable Bowel Syndrome

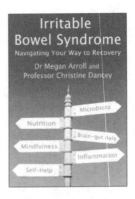

Irritable Bowel Syndrome
– navigating your way to recovery

By Dr Megan Arroll and Professor Christine Dancey
Print ISBN: 978-1-78161-069-5
Ebook ISBN: 978-1-78161-070-1

IBS is an 'invisible' disease – sufferers battle on pretending nothing is wrong and hiding their symptoms. Neither is it life-threatening. So nobody takes it seriously. But the authors do. This is a practical look at what we now know about the condition and all the latest approaches to treatment.

Sarah Stacey's Book of the Week, *You Magazine, Mail on Sunday*